Simply Relax

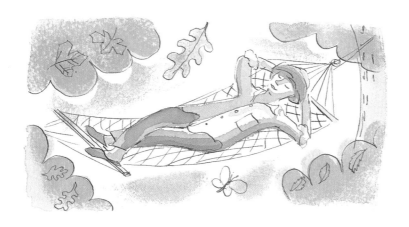

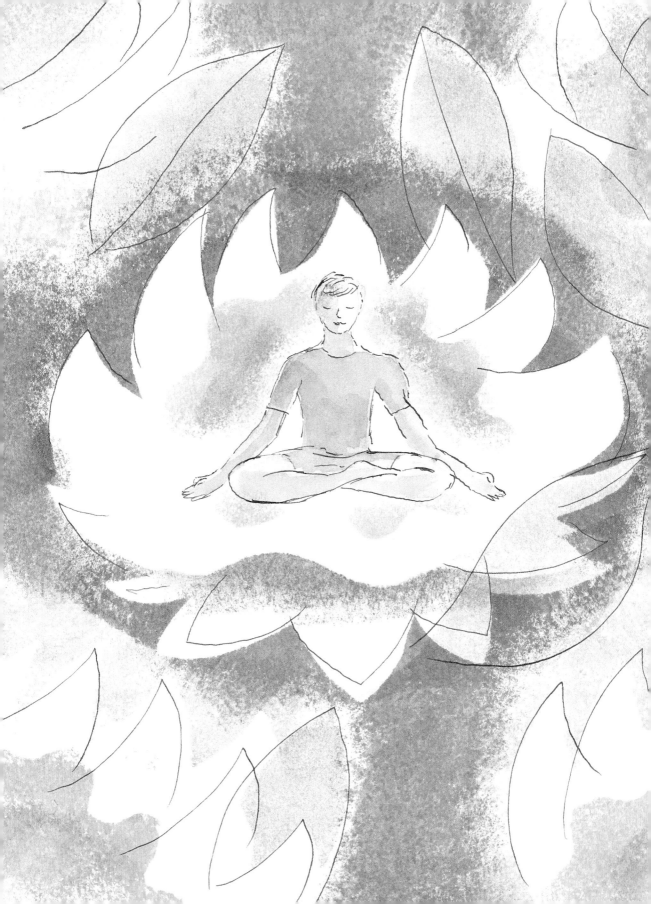

Simply Relax

The beginner's guide to relaxation

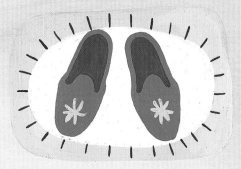

DR SARAH BREWER

DUNCAN BAIRD PUBLISHERS

LONDON

Simply Relax
Sarah Brewer

First published in the United Kingdom and Ireland in 2000 by
Duncan Baird Publishers Ltd
Sixth Floor, Castle House
75–76 Wells Street
London W1T 3QH

Conceived, created and designed by Duncan Baird Publishers

Managing Editor: Judy Barratt
Editors: Denise Alexander and Ingrid Court-Jones
Designers: Karen Wilks with Manisha Patel
Commissioned artwork: Allan Drummond and Katarzyna Klein

British Library Cataloguing-in-Publication Data:
A catalogue record for this book is available from the British Library

10 9 8 7 6 5 4 3

ISBN: 1-900131-29-3

Typeset in Bembo and Stone Sans
Colour reproduction by Colourscan, Singapore
Printed by Imago, Singapore

Publisher's Note
The Publishers and author recommend that medical advice is sought from your
own doctor before attempting any of the exercises or herbal or other treatments
suggested in this book. They can take no responsibility for any injury, damage or
other adverse effect resulting from following any of the suggestions herein.

Acknowledgment
Sarah Brewer would like to thank Toni Battison for her help with writing this book.

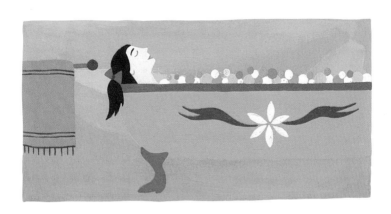

DEDICATION

For Richard and Saxon

Contents

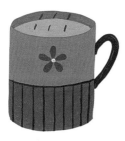
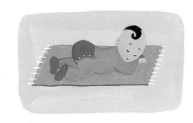
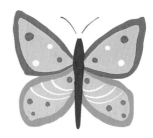

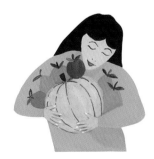
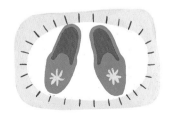
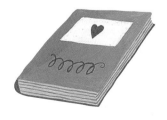

The Quest for Peace of Mind

In our high-tech and fast-paced world, our minds are always busy – we worry about our children, our finances and our social responsibilities. Perhaps we have to get used to new procedures at work or cope with our partner constantly being away on business. The opportunities for us to slow down, take our time, and finish things at our own pace are rare – for some of us they seem never to occur at all.

Learning to relax means finding the time for the important things in our lives – nurturing our inner selves, acquiring a positive attitude to life and, most of all, discovering peace of mind.

Simply Relax takes a holistic, practical and straight-forward approach to relaxation and shows a wealth of ways to simplify our lives and give us more time to enjoy the things that we love. In addition it shows us how to keep calm in a crisis, let the past go and move unburdened into the future, among many other things. By caring for our physical bodies, resting our minds and drawing on the healing power of the seasons, plants and animals, we can feel rejuvenated and see our problems in a new perspective. Along the way specially devised exercises deal with specific issues such as massage, or improving your self-confidence. Feel free to repeat the exercises as often as you like, or adapt them to fit with your lifestyle. The more you practise any relaxation exercise, the more effective it becomes.

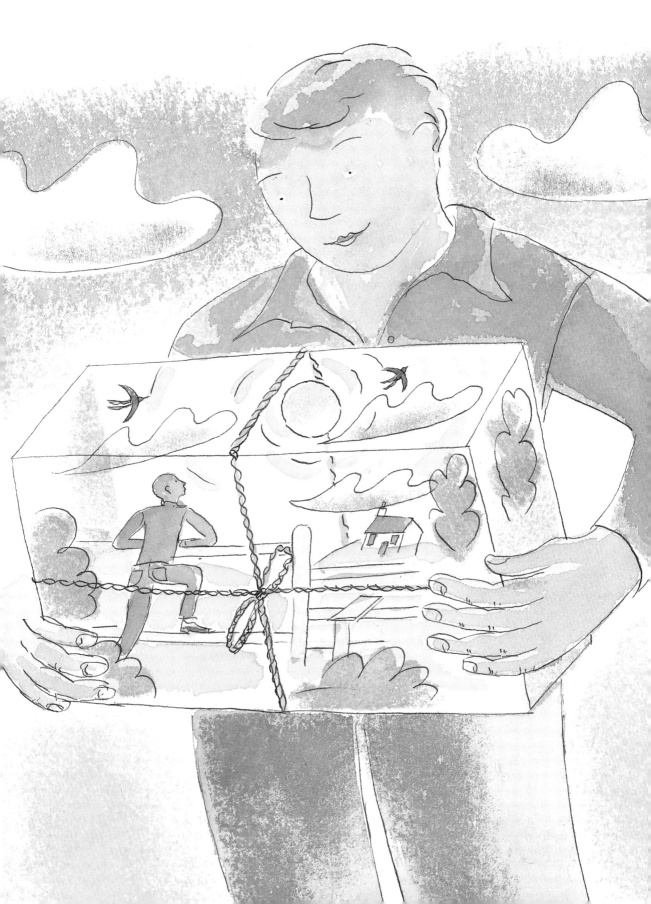

Bringing Relaxation Into Your Life

Relaxation is more than simply spending the weekend fishing, or taking two weeks out of the year to lie on a beach and bury ourselves in the pages of a good book. As valuable as taking a break from routine can be for short-term stress-relief, true relaxation comes only after we have learned to deal with life's natural flow, and restored the balance between body and mind, while following a few simple rules on the practicalities of living (such as eating healthily, taking gentle exercise and regulating our sleeping). This way we can begin to remove ourselves from the hectic pace of modern living and make relaxation an integral part of our lives.

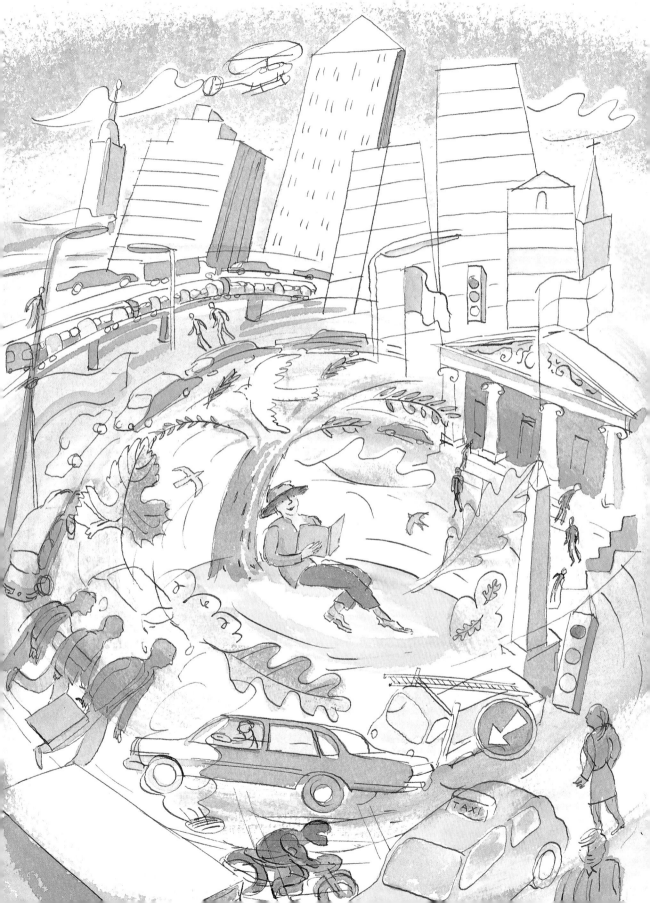

What is Stress?

We all need a little "spice" to keep us stimulated and interested in the world around us – the excitement of a vacation, the jubilation of a baby in the family, or the challenge of a new job. Without that spark life would soon lose its colour. Strictly speaking our daily responses to change or surprise are stress responses. When we become excited the hormone adrenaline (also known as epinephrine) turns on our alertness, helping us to focus on the event in hand. In straightforward, everyday circumstances there is certainly nothing untoward or harmful about its effects. Most of the time, however, when we talk of stress, we describe *distress* – the feelings we experience when tension is consistently high and adrenaline has been taking effect over a sustained period of time.

In the modern world we are under increasing, and often prolonged, pressure. But our physical reaction to stress developed thousands of years ago, and has changed very little since. In response to a perceived threat, we produce large amounts of adrenaline which causes our hearts to beat faster. This diverts more blood to the brain and muscles so we can think on our feet, fight or run away (known as the "fight or flight" reaction). This response was essential for primitive humans when confronted with a hostile wild animal, but is of much less use in the present day. For our ancestors the extra push was burned off, the adrenaline used up, and the body's natural balance soon restored. Nowadays we tend to experience stress under less energetic conditions, so that if we are, say, negotiating a business deal or moving home, we are unable to burn off our stress by running or fighting, and the adrenaline continues to build up in our bodies. Unless we take positive steps to release ourselves from its effects, we may develop harmful symptoms (see p.17), which can permanently damage our physical health and prey dangerously on our emotional well-being.

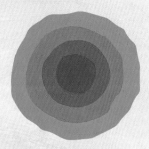

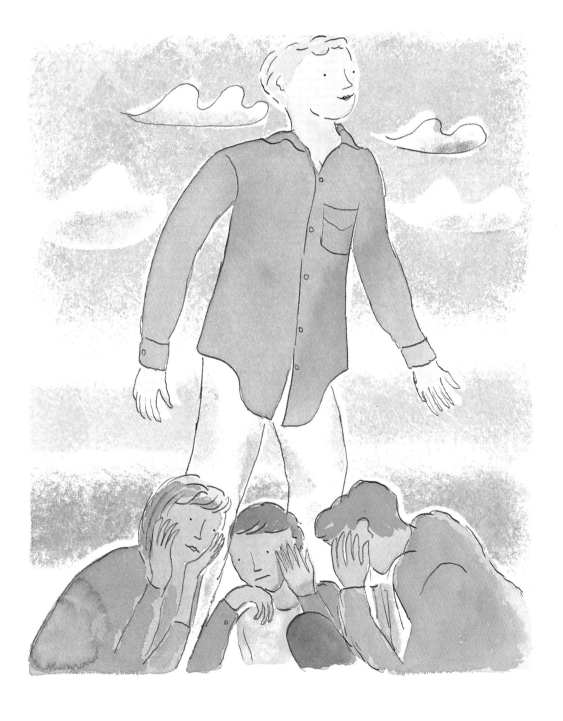

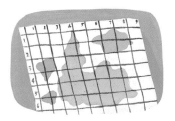

Relaxation prompts

Taking time out to have a break during times of stress is an effective way of renewing our energy. It may even allow us to find a solution to our problems. By developing a strategy for relaxation, so that we can guide ourselves into calm, we will be able to relax in even the most difficult of situations. Think of an activity that makes you feel calm: it may be a warm bath; a spell in the garden; or painting a picture. When you feel under excess pressure, take time out for your favourite relaxation activity, even if you don't feel like it initially. Your mind associates the pastime with relaxation so you will soon start to feel at peace.

The point at which healthy stress becomes distress varies for each of us. Imagine that you have a bag of stones slung over one shoulder. Each stone represents a worry, such as a difficult job or an unhappy relationship. The bag is so heavy that it threatens to throw you off balance and you have to keep putting it down. But, if you make an effort to stand tall, take regular breaks, distribute the load evenly and carry the bag squarely on your back, you will be able to complete your journey with far less discomfort. The same is true of stress. It is often not external events that make us feel overloaded or ill, but the way in which we cope with them.

The Greek philosopher Plato encapsulated what many people today have come to believe when he said "Nothing in the affairs of men is worthy of great anxiety." Bear this in mind as you frantically try to keep up with the pace of today's world – whatever stress is, it is not going to run or ruin your life. It is a demon that you can face and overcome – all that is needed is some perspective.

Before embarking upon a relaxation plan, try doing a stress assessment to identify the main difficulties in your life. Take a pen and paper and make a list of what events you believe have raised your stress levels recently – writing your concerns down will help you to clarify them in your mind. Perhaps a challenging boss has put you under extra pressure? Or your difficult teenage son or daughter has been particularly uncooperative this week? The items on your list don't have to be life-threatening – it's just as important to discern the relatively minor occurrences that cause you anxiety. How do you react to these situations? Is there anything practical you can do about them – look for a new job, or ask another family member to talk to your teenager? Stress is an enemy, but it is within your power to defeat it.

The Power of Qi

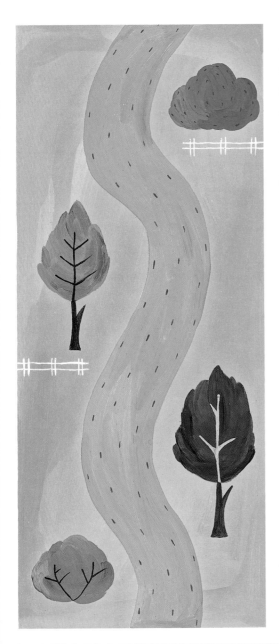

Chinese medicine teaches that physical, emotional and spiritual well-being depend upon the balance of qi energy in the body. Qi is an invisible life force that flows smoothly and abundantly through our systems when we are healthy. A healthy diet, regular sleep, tranquil thoughts and a calm approach to problems are all essential for good health.

Qi is believed to enter our body through the air we breathe and the food we eat, and we also have a supply of congenital qi, which is part of our genetic makeup. The aims of Chinese medicine, diet and martial arts are to maximize the flow of healthy qi in our bodies. According to the Chinese, abundant qi means that vitality and mental clarity can be retained throughout life and well into old age. It is the key to longevity.

Stress depletes our stores of qi and blocks its flow through the body, lowering our immunity to ill-health. There are many therapies that will help us release blocked qi. In acupuncture, for example, tiny needles are inserted into key points along the meridians (channels along which qi is said to flow through our bodies). By inserting these needles, acupuncturists believe that the movement of qi is released and regulated, restoring our bodies' natural balance.

Unmasking the Enemy

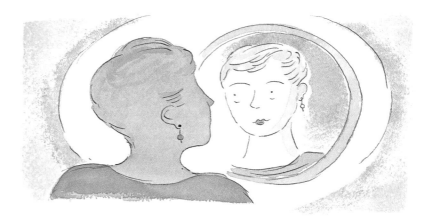

Initially, our symptoms of stress may be mild. If you find yourself sitting at your desk drumming your fingers, tapping your feet or biting your nails, or if you catch yourself frowning, you are probably feeling under pressure. Training ourselves to read these signs and take heed of them as soon as they appear is essential if we are to halt their metamorphosis into something more serious and disabling.

However, if such signs go unnoticed or, for whatever reasons, the early symptoms of stress are consciously ignored, the strain will begin to show itself in more obvious ways. Do your shoulders feel permanently tense? Do you feel so wound up after work that you need a couple of drinks just to switch off? Do you feel exhausted all the time? Or do you keep bursting into tears for no apparent reason? These are all signs that pressures are beginning to weigh heavily on your shoulders and urgent release is needed. You may try asking advice from a colleague, partner or counsellor; or you may prefer to sit down alone and try to identify exactly where the pressure comes from, then work out a strategy for its release. The only thing you should not do is ignore the problem – it will only get worse.

Although we all react in different ways to stress, symptoms generally fall into three categories: physical, mental and behavioural. These may appear separately or in combination and, to make matters worse, one set of symptoms is likely to lead to another. Our physical symptoms may cause mental difficulties, such as depression, and in turn, lead to behavioural problems, such as avoiding our friends and relations. It is equally likely that, if our mental health shows signs of strain, such as listlessness and negativity, physical symptoms are hot on their heels.

The symptoms each of us shows can be unique, so it is important that we listen to our own bodies. Stress can affect any part of us, but in most cases, it manifests itself in one area. Does your skin break out just before an important date? Does your head begin to throb at the first sign of trouble? Does an old sporting injury begin to twinge when you have a job interview? Do you always come down with a cold before a vacation? If you become aware of your body, these habitual symptoms of stress may act as valuable warning signs that trouble is building up. You may not have realized how much pressure you are taking on, but a severe attack of indigestion, or a migraine that forces you to retire to your bed, will let you know that your body and mind are coming under increasing strain. In general, physical symptoms are caused by the "fight or flight" changes in our bodies (see p.12). The instinctive nature of these physical changes means that we may exhibit symptoms before we consciously realize that we are under pressure.

Once physical symptoms appear, they may remain for some time. Imagine that you are like a piece of elastic. You are constantly stretched and released. For a while, you can snap back into your original state and not show any ill effects. But if the stress continues and you are stretched again and again, you begin to show signs of wear and tear, you become worn and not so elastic. If you don't take action, you may snap in two – becoming seriously ill or suffering a breakdown. Everyone reaches breaking point at a different time (see p.14), and only you can know if stress is beginning to take its toll.

As well as physical signs of stress, we are equally vulnerable to emotional symptoms (mental symptoms that often manifest

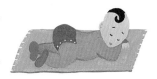

Symptoms checklist

The following list gives some physical, emotional and behavioural symptoms of stress. If you find you are regularly troubled by more than five of them, it is time to take action.

- *headaches*
- *tiredness and listlessness*
- *sleeplessness*
- *palpitations and rapid pulse*
- *indigestion or heart burn*
- *breathing problems*
- *aching joints*
- *over- or under-eating*
- *smoking or drinking too much*
- *skin problems*
- *increased urine output and nervous diarrhoea*
- *numbness and pins and needles*
- *poor concentration and difficulty making decisions*
- *unhappiness or depression*
- *feelings of anger, frustration or helplessness*
- *feelings of irritability or tearfulness*
- *anxiousness and fearfulness*
- *being without a sense of humour*

themselves behaviourally). We may begin to feel insecure or paranoid, doubt the love we receive from our family, or find it hard to believe our superiors when we are praised. These are all warning signs that we need to take positive steps to unburden ourselves. We may need to ask for help or force ourselves to take a break.

The greater our feelings of despair or our physical discomfort, the more we seek to relieve them. We may change our behaviour to mask our problems or avoid the issues that cause us concern. These strategies, far from resolving the stress, are often the most obvious indicators to our family, friends and colleagues that our problems are becoming too much. Do you attempt to solve your sleeping problems by drinking alcohol at night? Do you find yourself reaching for chocolate after an argument with your partner? Do you try to avoid confronting your boss by working from home on days when he or she is in the office?

By conquering our symptoms, we can tackle the source of our stress with more efficiency. A regular meditation may help you begin to combat stress. Set aside ten minutes every morning, perhaps before breakfast, for yourself. You might want to go into the garden, if you have one, or a quiet room. Make sure you are sitting or standing comfortably. Take a few deep breaths and make yourself aware of your body – you might notice that your heart is racing, your muscles are tense or there are constant thoughts running around your head. Say "stop" to yourself and visualize all of the symptoms of stress disappearing. Replace them with a feeling of calm and warmth, think of your heart rate as a slow, steady beat, imagine your muscles loosening and lengthening. If you do this each morning, you will begin the day in a calm and positive frame of mind and you will notice more readily stress symptoms that crop up.

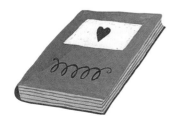

Exercise 1
Keeping a Stress Diary

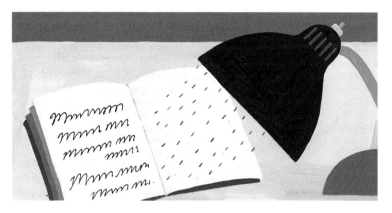

Sometimes, although we may recognize a symptom of stress, it can be hard to identify the cause. Keeping a stress diary will help you to identify the causes and patterns of stress symptoms so that you can make helpful changes in your life.

• Use a blank notebook or diary. Begin by keeping it for a week, and then extend it if you feel the trigger-symptom patterns have not revealed themselves. Divide each page horizontally into sections – for example: "bed to work"; "morning"; "afternoon"; "evening to bed."

• Fill in your diary as often as you can – preferably as each stress symptom occurs. Note down precisely what happened just before it appeared. Also jot down all your activities and how you were feeling at the time, even if no symptom was apparent. Are any patterns emerging?

• At the end of the first week, take a look at when you felt stressed and when you were relaxed. You may notice that you felt most under pressure when shopping – try to go at a quieter time. If you felt relaxed during evenings with your children, try to spend more time with them. Soon the stress journal will guide your life onto a quieter path.

Regaining Calm

Going with the flow

According to the Chinese philosophy of Daoism, life has a natural flow. Just as the water in a river collects debris from the banks as it weaves its meandering course, so our lives pick up objects (in the form of responsibilities, habits and experiences) as we move through time. In order to regain calm, we should try to learn that obstacles can never halt our flow: we can always find a course around them. Whenever you feel yourself trying to push one of life's obstacles out of the way, let go of your effort. Think of ways to work around it and revel in the sense of release this attitude gives.

Relaxation is a healing process – a remedy to combat the effects of stress and restore the balance between mind and body. By turning our attention inwards, it is possible to regain calm and tune in to the body's rhythms. If we learn to relax by putting in place long-term coping strategies, as well as identifying quick-fix relaxation techniques for times of heightened pressure, there is no need to blot out life's problems with temporary measures such as drinking, smoking or taking drugs – stimulants which ultimately cause us a great deal of harm.

One of the most common responses to stress is to "bury our heads in the sand" (pretend that our anxieties are not there). However, without proper release, tension builds up in our muscles and our minds, making us stiff and inflexible, physically and mentally, and therefore more prone to stress. Dealing with stress requires positive action and only once we have removed the built-up layers of stress in our current lives can we look at ways of maintaining inner peace. Begin by making a conscious effort to slow down. Even if you are in an environment where deadlines need to be met, try to create an action plan for time management (see p.122). Remember the cautionary tale of the hare who raced off at a very fast pace, but soon ran out of steam and was beaten to the finishing line by the gentle-paced tortoise.

Another tentative first step is to begin to identify the day-to-day things that make us anxious. Among them might be jostling for a place on the bus during rush-hour or standing in line at the supermarket. Try to identify practical solutions to these daily situations (perhaps going to the preceding bus stop or doing the shopping soon after the store opens); or put them into perspective and aim to detach yourself from them (see p.68); or see them in a positive light: for example, standing in line could give us quiet time for contemplation.

Exercise 2
Whole Body Relaxation

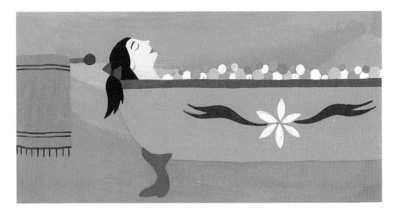

One of the best ways to relax physically is to find somewhere warm and quiet to lie down and concentrate on releasing tension in each of the muscle groups. If you like, you could try this exercise as you soak in a warm bath.

• Close your eyes. Lift your arms into the air, bending them at the elbow and clenching your fists. Breathe in deeply; then, as you breathe out, release your clenched fists. Lower your arms gently and imagine the tension in them draining away. Your fingers may even start to tingle.

• Now shrug your shoulders as high as you can. Feel the tension in your head, shoulders, neck and chest. Hold for a moment; then, on an out-breath, slowly release. Imagine the tension flowing away. Tighten your facial muscles by screwing up your face and clenching your teeth. Hold for a few seconds, then let go.

• Continue working through your muscles, tensing and releasing in this way, paying particular attention to your back, abdomen, buttocks and legs. Once you are done, a feeling of warmth should wash over you and your body should feel completely calm and relaxed.

Healthy Living

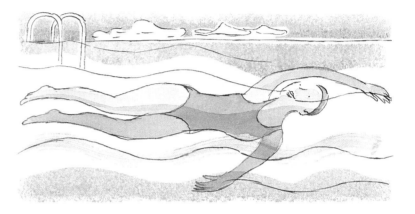

When we find ourselves juggling each different aspect of our lives – our work, our families and our friends, to name but a few – we often find that, in order to keep all the balls in the air, we compromise the most straightforward and practical ways we have of achieving well-being for ourselves. For example, how many times have you thought to yourself that you really should do some exercise, and then in the same moment banished the idea as preposterous – where would you find the time? How often have you promised yourself that you will go to bed earlier, and then found that midnight has come and gone and you are only just turning in for the night?

Many of us make solemn vows to ourselves about improving our general living habits, knowing that we can reap great benefits to our health and daily productivity by doing so, only to dismiss such ideas because we feel we haven't the time or are too tired or distracted to carry them out. However, basic living patterns – the quality of our waking time, how well we sleep (see p.50) and what we eat and drink – form the foundations that hold up the rest of our lives, and set the levels of healthiness at which we live.

One of the first things to falter when stress begins to take hold is exercise. Our bodies are designed for activity, not for the sedentary lifestyle that many of us have adopted today. In order to benefit from regular exercise, we don't need to start going to high-impact aerobics classes or take up a competitive sport. Low-impact exercise, such as walking or swimming, even for as little as ten minutes a day, can improve our general fitness many times over. Exercise forces us to take time out for ourselves, encouraging us to become absorbed in something other than our daily pressures; and it is a form of inner self-massage: as our muscles stretch, they release tension built up over a busy day. Some exercise teachers believe that stressful experiences become locked in parts of our bodies. For example, an upsetting row with your partner or a work colleague might cause the muscles in, say, your shoulders to become tight. Exercise releases this tension, and the subject of discussion is set free, allowing us to perceive it with renewed clarity or to be released from it altogether. In addition, during physical activity our breathing becomes deeper and more rhythmic, massaging our lungs and diaphragm and letting go of stress with each out-breath.

The saying "you are what you eat" is increasingly known to be true. Every building block in the body is ultimately derived from our food, which must provide all the vitamins, minerals, fibre, essential fatty acids, protein and energy needed for optimum health. And yet when time becomes our enemy we often find ourselves reaching for fast food (sometimes even delivered to our doorstep) and quick snacks, which are rustled up in a matter of minutes and often lacking in any true nutritious value. Even worse, we might skip meals altogether.

For optimum nutrition we might try following the old adage that it is best to breakfast like a king, lunch like a prince and dine like a pauper. As clichéd as it sounds, breakfast *is* the most important meal of the day. It helps to boost blood sugar levels and kick-start the metabolism. Missing breakfast often means that our concentration is

Feeling fit

It does not take a drastic change to your lifestyle to become fit. If you can spare an hour or so a week, try gentle jogging through a park or swimming. Alternatively, you might cycle to work instead of taking the train. Include exercise in your daily life: take the stairs instead of the lift, walk to fetch a newspaper or sandwich for lunch; even getting off the bus one or two stops earlier and walking the rest of the way to work or back home provides regular, beneficial exercise and eats only minimally into our time.

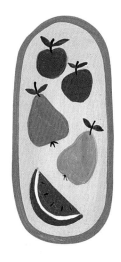

poor and that we become easily irritable – and, if we start the day stressed, the likelihood is that our unease and discomfort will only build up over the following hours.

Ideally, lunch should be the biggest meal of the day. Around lunchtime, the metabolism is happily ticking away, turning what we eat into the energy that will see us through the afternoon. Many nutritionists suggest that it is best to avoid fatty foods (for example, fried foods, or cakes and sweets) over lunch, which some studies have shown can make us sluggish in the afternoon. Eat a snack in the mid afternoon and try to keep your dinners light. Our digestive systems can process a small amount of food much more efficiently before we retire to bed than one large meal at the end of the day.

The healthiest diet is one that is low in harmful, unsaturated fats and high in grains, pulses, fruit and vegetables. Animal and dairy products are regarded as extremely nourishing, but only in small quantities. If eaten in excess, such products are believed to upset digestion and the overall balance of health.

The ancient Greek physician Hippocrates declared "Let food be your medicine and medicine be your food." Green and yellow fruit and vegetables contain protective substances that boost the immune system, keeping our bodies and our minds strong and healthy. Fresh fruit and vegetables contain vitamins, including B-complex vitamins and vitamin C, that are essential for good health. Unfortunately, these important nutrients are rapidly used up by the body during times of stress. Emotional props, such as smoking cigarettes, eating sugary comfort foods or drinking excess alcohol can increase feelings of tension as well as deplete these vitamin levels further. Replenishing your body's nutritional supplies will help you to deal with unease.

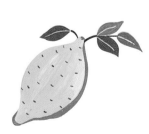

The Mediterranean Diet

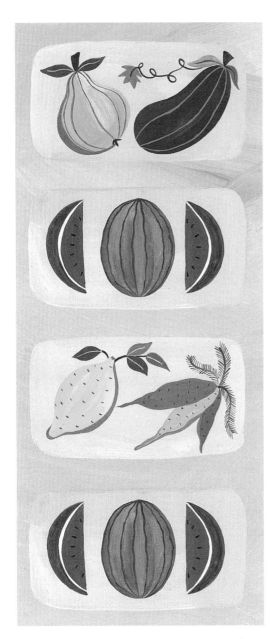

According to the World Health Organization, one of the most nutritious diets in the world is that adopted by the people of the Mediterranean, such as those of Italy, eastern Spain, the south of France and Greece. It is no coincidence that, in these regions, cases of heart disease are the lowest in Europe.

On a Mediterranean diet at least half our daily food intake should be made up of carbohydrates, such as bread, pasta and cereals. These will provide us with energy and fibre, which helps digestion. Next, we should eat plenty of seasonal fresh fruit and vegetables. We need a minimum of five servings of these every day for vital vitamins and minerals. A serving could be an apple, a small salad or a baked potato. Protein and fats – in the form of white meat, oily fish, pulses and unsaturated vegetable oils – should make up the remaining small, but nonetheless vital, component of our diets. Protein and fat promote growth and give us the energy we need every day.

Eating Mediterranean-style is a leisurely and often sociable affair. It makes sense, therefore, to take your time over meals, and savour the rich diversity of flavours in each mouthful, while enjoying the pleasant company of family and friends.

Self-belief

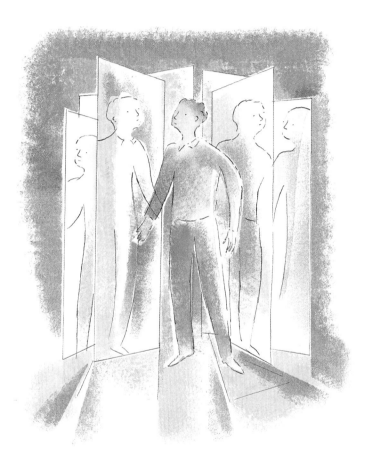

Self-belief is an essential step on the road to relaxation. But it is often difficult to think in a positive and self-nurturing way when we feel under pressure. Psychological studies have shown that one of the most common self-perceptions among all human beings is "I am not good enough." Whatever the root of the self-doubt (be it a repressed childhood or highly competitive peers), low self-esteem is unquestionably one of the greatest causes of stress – it performs exactly the opposite of its intention (to reduce fear of failure by starting out with low expectations), because inevitably any negative experiences only confirm our perceived right to be unhappy with ourselves. Even if we achieve something positive, we tend to pass it off as a lucky twist of fate, rather than an encouraging affirmation of our abilities. In contrast, if we have confidence in ourselves, we exude an aura that produces positive emotions and events in our lives. We are able to relate to others in a more fulfilling way and we become magnets for success.

To build up our self-confidence, we need begin in only small ways. Try to adopt the habit of praising yourself for any successes, even if they seem slight. For example, if you have fulfilled a promise to yourself to get up in time to have a proper breakfast, give yourself a reward: if it is a sunny morning, eat in the garden, enjoying the fresh air. Make a conscious effort to substitute positive thoughts for negative ones: "I am not good enough" then becomes "I am good enough." Once you get into the habit of catching yourself when you say negative things, and replacing them as often as you can, you will soon be able automatically to make positive affirmations in any given situation. In the event of an emotional crisis, they will have a profoundly calming effect. The word "calm" in itself can also act as a *mantra* (see p.42) – repeating it to yourself can help you to relax in times of stress.

Many of us tend to be embarrassed by compliments – we feel awkward that someone else views us (or something about us) in a more positive light than we view ourselves. If someone offers you praise, make a conscious effort simply to thank them – try not to rationalize what they have said, or to undo it, just accept it.

Try to avoid comparing yourself with others. We all know people who seem more successful than we are, but each of us has different strengths and weaknesses, different paces by which to work and methods by which to get things done. Make an effort to believe in your own ways: it is much harder and more unfulfilling to try to follow someone else's logic than it is to trust in our own. This is rather like trying to drive to a destination using our partner's route rather than the one we would use by ourselves. We will probably take longer to get where we are going, and we are certainly more liable to get lost!

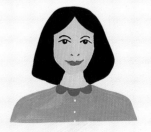

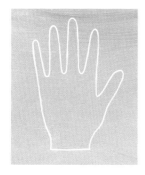

Remember that a mistake is not a catastrophe. It is unrealistic to think that we can be right all the time, and it does not automatically follow that one error of judgement will trigger a whole series of mistakes. If you have made an error, take responsibility for it, do all you can to rectify it, and then let it go. We need strength of character to own up to our mistakes, but by doing so we will feel better about ourselves, and others will respect our honesty and efforts.

One tell-tale sign of low self-esteem is the inability to assert ourselves calmly and articulately. For some of us, asserting even small needs, such as having to cancel a dinner with a friend, wracks us with guilt. Even more so, we may find that asking our boss for a pay rise or help during busy times fills us with dread.

Calm articulation of our problems releases burdens from our shoulders. Even if no successful conclusion is reached, expressing our requests clearly can make us feel more confident – we may not be able to persuade someone to see things our way, but we have been true to ourselves. Think about how pleased with yourself you have felt when you have been open and honest about a difficult topic; or what an enormous relief it felt to say "no" (politely, of course) to more work when you already felt that you were overburdened.

There are also many other ways to train ourselves to be more assertive, and so increase our self-belief. Make sure that you have a clear idea of the compromises that you can make. If assertiveness is not in your nature, break yourself in gently. At first, try to reach a conclusion that gives you the minimum you are willing to accept. As you become more confident, see if you can arrive at a decision that fulfils your original goal, but always be prepared to meet on middle ground. Riding roughshod rarely helps anyone – least of all ourselves.

Exercise 3
Taking the Podium of Success

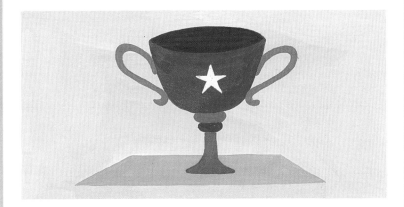

One of the best ways to begin to believe in ourselves is to create a combined visualization-affirmation around potential achievement. The following exercise aims to instil in your consciousness that success is always within your grasp.

• Every night before you fall asleep, close your eyes and visualize yourself receiving an award (it may be related to a specific goal, or be simply for being a good friend, a reliable employee or a loving partner). The crowd is cheering and smiling. You are filled with pride.

• Imagine turning to face the crowd, holding your award firmly with both hands. Visualize the flash of cameras and the excited faces in the throng below you. Now repeat an affirmation to yourself (and to the crowd in your imagination): it can be general, such as "I am a winner!" or something more specific, such as "I am no longer scared of flying."

• Repeat the affirmation ten times. Each time you say it, imagine lifting your award high into the air to an enormous cheer from the crowd. In a few days and nights, the affirmation will begin to take root in your consciousness, and the seeds of your success will be sown.

Summing Up

- If something triggers stress – take time out. Relax. Give yourself a break!

- Have an emergency relaxation plan for when things get tough – soak in a bath or take a walk until you feel calm.

- Take care of your body. It will see you through the toughest of times.

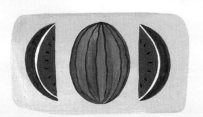 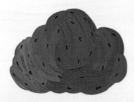 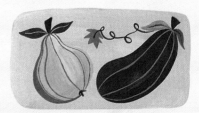

- Remind yourself of your successes. Be proud of what you've achieved.

- In every situation, try to surround yourself in a blissful oasis of tranquillity – nothing can get you down.

- Stress is weak without you! It cannot run or ruin your life – you are strong.

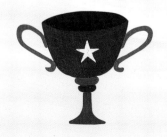 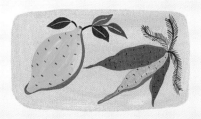 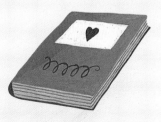

Body and Mind in Harmony

The ancient Greek philosopher Plato taught that if the body is to be healthy, we must begin by curing the mind. This was accepted wisdom until the seventeenth century, when modern medicine deliberately separated the studies of mind and body. In the present day, the pendulum has swung back, and more and more of us are recognizing that we cannot be truly healthy unless we nourish our minds as well as our bodies. We seek a holistic approach to health and relaxation – one that considers our mental and physical health in harmony. As a result a wide range of alternative therapies from both East and West that appeal to our senses, and emphasize the value of relaxation and rejuvenating sleep, are once again gaining in popularity.

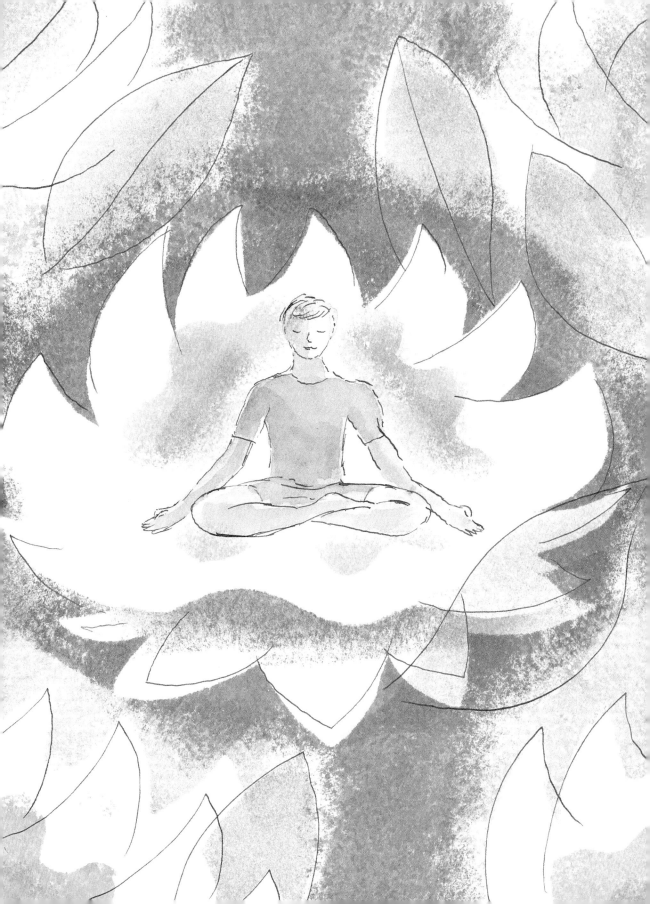

Finding Balance

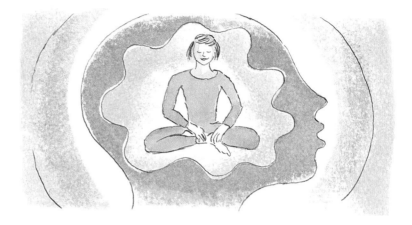

Just as stress affects our mental and physical health (see p.17), relaxation, to be effective, must calm our racing minds as well as soothe our tense bodies. If we can learn to balance our mind and body, we can learn to recognize imbalances when they occur. In this way, we repair ourselves in the present, and arm ourselves for the future.

The holistic principles of Eastern therapeutic medicine are ideal for true relaxation. Perhaps the most popular and simple to practise alone are meditation and yoga. In meditation we still our minds, allowing our inherent inner peace to flow through our bodies and ease away tension. Yoga gently stretches and moves our bodies as we breathe deeply and slowly, focusing our minds on the gentle movement and calming us through the deep breathing. Countless scientific experiments have shown the profound beneficial effects of both these techniques on blood pressure, stiff joints, heart rate and muscular tension, as well as on depression, fatigue and anxiety.

For centuries religions all over the world have used meditation to aid the contemplation of the divine godhead – but you don't have to be religious to reap its benefits. Find a quiet place to sit where you are unlikely to be disturbed. (When you are more experienced you will be able to "switch off" and meditate in the busiest of environments, such as on a train or in the middle of a crowd of people.) Sit cross-legged on the floor, or in a straight-backed chair with both your feet flat on the floor. Your back should be straight and poised but not rigid. Make sure that you are comfortable. Close your eyes and take a few deep breaths, taking care to breathe from your abdomen and not from your chest (see p.38). Focus your thoughts on a mental image, perhaps your favourite flower or your partner's face, or silently chant a word, such as "calm", "peace" or "one". Every time your mind begins to wander, gently bring yourself back to your word or image. You may be surprised at how undisciplined your thoughts are at first, but with practice you will be able to remain focused for as long as you like. When you first begin meditation, practise the exercise for about five minutes, gradually increasing to twenty minutes or half an hour. Those who meditate daily find that they are able to tap easily into profound calm during otherwise difficult or stressful times. Furthermore, the calm experienced during an early morning meditation remains all through the day.

Mediation and yoga go hand in hand. Throughout the practice of yoga, the mind should remain focused as in meditation. Although it is best to learn yoga from a qualified teacher, try doing the following basic *asana* (posture) once a day – perhaps each morning when you wake up. Stand up straight, both feet firmly on the floor, close your eyes and breathe slowly for a few minutes. Then, keeping your breathing calm and rhythmic, gently lift both your arms in front of your body and up so that your hands are reaching high over your head toward the sky. Hold the stretch for about a minute. As you do so, be aware of your body: feel your feet pressing into the ground; feel the muscles in your limbs; notice the position of your head and enjoy the stretch of your spine. Imagine that you are drawing calming, positive energy from the sun. Focus your mind on visualizing this energy entering your outstretched fingertips and coursing through your body, invigorating you for the day ahead. Slowly bring your arms down by your sides, and shake them gently. You feel revitalized, in balance and at peace.

Time to relax

The best way to benefit from meditation and yoga is to set aside a certain time every day to practise them. Some people find the early morning works best: we are calm after a night's sleep and the issues of the day have not yet invaded our minds. The dawn is traditionally the time when the spirit world and the earthly world meet, and is therefore conducive to meditation and altered states of consciousness.

Others find it beneficial to set aside time after work, separating the toils of the day from the activities of the evening. Meditation or yoga at the end of the day cleanses us of work irritations and prepares us for time with our families and friends. Spend a few minutes now deciding on the best time at which you can practise regular contemplation. Once relaxation becomes part of your everyday routine, stress will be pushed out.

The Art of Breathing

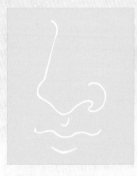

Breathing is the key to life. As we breathe, oxygen nourishes every cell in our bodies, helping to keep us healthy. Breathing is very closely connected to our state of mind. When life is peaceful and we are free from tension, we breathe calmly, deeply and regularly. But when stress levels rise, our breathing becomes fast, shallow and irregular.

Most of us tend not to breathe properly. Years of stress or worry have made shallow, fast breathing (in extreme cases this is called hyperventilation, or over-breathing) seem normal. In general, we use only the top third of our lungs to take in air. Is your chest moving up and down when you breathe? Is your abdomen almost still? You may not be using your lungs properly. Along with poor habits such as deep sighs, gasps and breath-holding, incorrect breathing causes an imbalance in the oxygen and carbon dioxide levels circulating around the body. Toxins aren't breathed out properly, and we become tired and susceptible to illness – the last thing we need during times of stress. Hyperventilation is one of the main causes of panic attacks, and if it persists over a long period of time, may cause frightening symptoms, such as chest pain, numbness, muscle spasm and even total collapse.

Quite simply, if we learn to breathe properly we can improve the quality of our lives. Try a visualization exercise to see how well you can breathe. Sit comfortably, loosen your clothing, and close your eyes. Imagine a gently flickering candle in front of you. In your mind's eye, focus on it as you inhale and exhale and try to push other thoughts out of your mind. As you breathe in, imagine that the candle flame is sucked toward you – the deeper the in-breath, the more pronounced the flame's direction. As you breathe out in a long, slow exhalation, the flame bends away. The aim is not to blow out the imaginary candle, but to cause it to flicker away from you as far as you can. Continue to

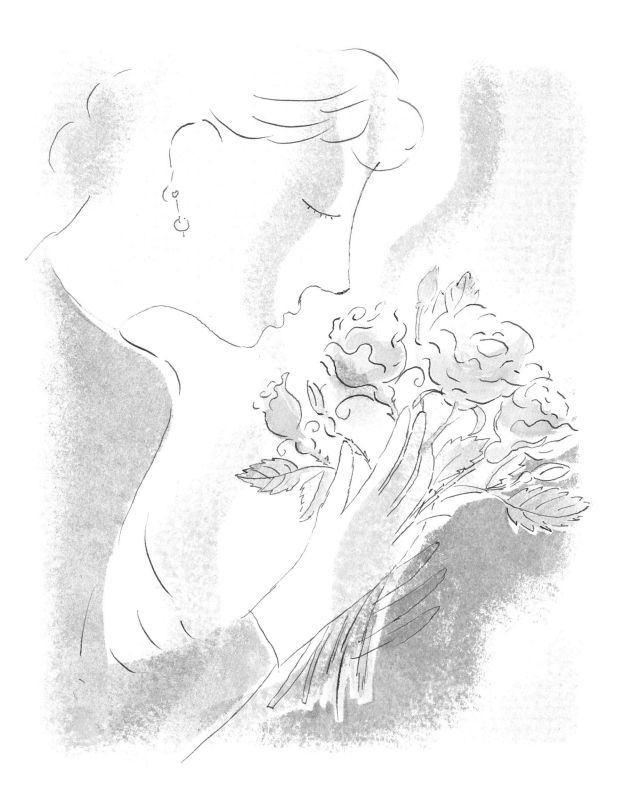

breathe like this, but place one hand on your abdomen and the other on your upper chest. If you are breathing correctly, as you inhale, your lower hand should rise far more than your upper hand. How fast are you breathing? The in- and out-breath cycle should take five seconds.

Yoga can also help us to relax and breathe properly. Find a quiet place where you have room to stretch. Stand comfortably with your legs slightly more than a shoulder-width apart and your feet facing forward. As you slowly breathe in, raise your right arm alongside your right ear. Stretch as high as possible. As you breathe out, bend to the right, so that your body forms a graceful curve from your fingertips to your feet. Breathe regularly and hold the position for at least 30 seconds. Make sure that you keep looking forwards, not down; that your knees and upper elbow are straight; and that your body and feet are not twisted. Inhale as you return to the starting position. Repeat the exercise, this time using the left arm and moving to the left.

In times of acute stress, taking a moment to slow our breathing will instantly calm us. Next time you are under pressure, take a break, and imagine lying on a warm beach on a beautiful island in the middle of the ocean. Listen to the waves lazily lapping against the shore. Notice the pattern of your breathing and try to harmonize it with the ebb and flow of the waves, until they become as one – your breathing is relaxed, calm and attuned with the rhythm of the water.

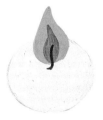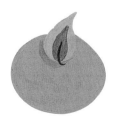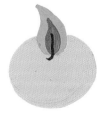

Exercise 4
The Complete Breath

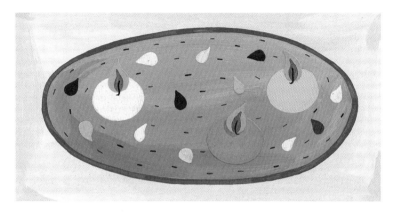

The relationship between our breathing patterns and state of mind lies at the core of meditation and yoga practices. The Complete Breath is a useful pranayama (yogic breath control) exercise that will calm and soothe the mind.

• Remove your shoes and loosen your clothing. Lie down, either on the floor or on a bed, making sure that there is plenty of room above your head. Let your arms relax at your sides.

• Close your eyes and inhale very slowly through your nose. Breathe out slowly through your nose – ideally your out-breath should take twice as long as your in-breath. Breathe this way for a minute or two until you feel calm.

• When you feel ready, breathe in slowly and at the same time raise your arms above your head. As you do this imagine your lungs expanding and filling with pure, nourishing air.

• Slowly breathe out, lower your arms to your sides and relax. Repeat the sequence as many times as you like.

The Power of Touch

Quick-fix through touch

Practise the following technique when you are already feeling relaxed, and then you can call upon it as a relaxation trigger whenever you are stressed. Sit in a quiet place, and touch the tip of your thumb with the index finger on the same hand. Think back to a time when you felt happy and relaxed: a birthday party when you were very young; or when you held your child for the first time. Imagine the scene in as much detail as you can. Allow the positive emotions of that time to wash through you, then imagine them converging at the point where your finger and thumb touch. The next time you are feeling tense, touch your thumb with the same finger, and imagine the blissful feelings of your visualization are being released from the point of contact to flood through your body.

Imagine life if you couldn't feel another living thing. Studies have shown that without physical contact with other living beings, we are more likely to become sick, depressed and anxious. Touch does not necessarily mean sexual contact: just a hand placed over ours or a brief squeeze of our shoulder connects us with the people around us and can reassure and calm us; a hug from a friend can let us know how much we are cared for and appreciated.

When we are newborn babies, suddenly expelled from the cozy security of the womb, we need constant reassurance from our mother and close contact with the warmth of her body. As we grow up we learn that touch is fundamental to survival – from the simple action of withdrawing from pain, to keeping our footing on a slippery surface. The sense of touch enriches, eases or offers protection during every moment of our lives.

Not surprisingly, using touch is a very effective way of ensuring that we remain relaxed. A number of holistic therapies have evolved around this very important sense. Healers often work by laying their hands on people, and massage is not only one of the most popular methods of relaxation, it is among the basic techniques of Chinese, Ayurvedic and Japanese traditional medicines.

Although massage is usually practised with a partner, self-massage can also relieve symptoms of stress, such as a headache or eye strain, and promote tranquillity. Using gentle pressure, smooth the tips of your fingers over your forehead, working from the centre out to your temples. Repeat this several times. Next, using the palms of your hands, fingers pointing horizontally across your brow, smooth up toward your hairline, one hand after the other. Repeat this movement ten times or until you feel all your tension draining away.

Exercise 5
A Soothing Massage

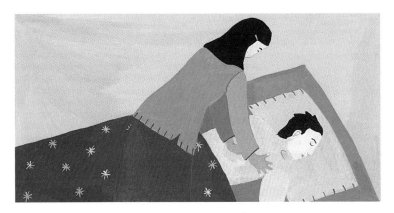

In times of stress our neck and shoulders often become stiff and painful. Giving and receiving a soothing massage will help both the masseur and the person being massaged to relax physically and mentally.

• Make sure the room is warm, and set the scene with soft candlelight and relaxing music. Choose a firm but comfortable surface for the massage – for example, several towels spread on the floor.

• Ask your partner to undress and lie down. Place a few drops of massage oil into your palms and knead the skin around your partner's shoulder blade. After a few minutes, repeat on the other shoulder.

• Place your hands between the tops of the shoulder blades, and, using light pressure, massage in small circles with your thumbs. Work down the spine a little and follow the line of the shoulder blades outward.

• Place your hands on the right shoulder, and gently, but firmly, squeeze the muscle between your thumb and fingers. Continue until you feel all muscle stiffness releasing. Repeat on the other side.

Harmony and Song

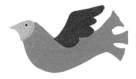

More than 2,000 years ago, Epictetus the Stoic noted "God gave man two ears, but only one mouth, that he might hear twice as much as he speaks." Our hearing is not only the process that facilitates communication through sound, but it also provides a direct channel to our spirit. Think about how moved we can be by a passage of music (even pieces of music without special association for us), or the comfort we find in the sound of a familiar and friendly voice. With so many positive associations, sound makes a perfect focus for relaxation.

In Hindu philosophy, during his primeval meditation, the creator-god Brahma uttered a sacred sound, and this created the universe. This sound is known as a *mantra* and is made up of phrases or a single syllable (such as *Om*). Repeated gently during meditation, a mantra is said to focus and calm the mind. Both mantras and Gregorian chants, with their soothing, repetitive, harmonious notes and extended vowels, appeal to the creative right side of the brain, and can be used to raise levels of consciousness, and to produce many physical and emotional effects. When singing in harmony, for example, the pupils of our eyes dilate and our brains produce natural relaxation chemicals.

Even if you think that you are unable to sing in tune, singing in the bath or shower or in the car on the way to work, for example, can be profoundly relaxing – it releases tension and, importantly, encourages us to breathe deeply and rhythmically.

The sounds of nature can present us with a harmonious focus for meditation. Try taking an early morning walk through a park. Sit on a bench or on the grass, close your eyes, and try to distinguish as many different sounds as you can. Perhaps you can hear children playing, the buzzing of a bee collecting nectar, or the sound of the wind through the trees. Try to focus on extending your hearing as far as you can.

Exercise 6
Tuning into Relaxation

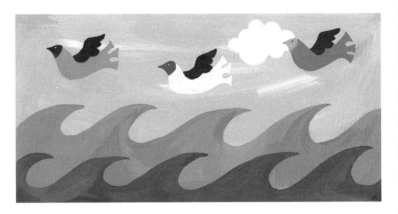

Creating your own relaxation tape is a perfect way to let sound ease your troubles away – even if the tape is not at hand one day, you can play it over in your head for inner peace.

• Choose some soft, quiet music that appeals to you. Perhaps a favourite classical piece, a slow song, or a tune that reminds you of your childhood. Make sure the music lasts for at least ten minutes.

• If you can, try recording some sounds from nature onto your tape – perhaps the sound of the sea, the sound of a stream or birds singing – whatever you find relaxing and pleasant to listen to.

• Once you have recorded all that you want to, play the tape as you lie comfortably in a warm, private room. Tune your breath into the music's rhythm or the sound of nature. Separate the sounds and then let them merge into one.

• Listen to the tape at least once a day – once you know it well, you will be able to call upon it in your mind any time you like.

Vision and Colour

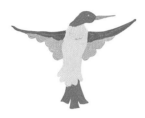

The energy of light

In order to see we need light. The idea of a powerful light energy has been recognized for thousands of years.

Every morning the sun's light stimulates us and revives us; and its absence prompts us to sleep. Light energy is so vitalizing, that when we want to relax, we often close our eyes first. Make a mental note of how your body and emotions react to changing light. Use the information you glean to better understand your body's rhythms – promise to live by them as much as you can.

It is mainly through our sense of sight that we appraise the world around us. However, all too often we take for granted what we can see. Bring to mind a journey that you regularly make by foot – it might be from your home to the nearest store, or from the train station to your place of work. Make the journey in your mind's eye, taking it slowly and carefully. As you do so note down all the things that you pass on the way – the colours of the flowers in your neighbour's garden, the architecture of the houses, callboxes on the sidewalk, the sign outside your office building. When you next make the journey, see how accurate your mind's eye has been – what were the things that you missed altogether? Did you imagine the colours differently?

Most of us carry out our daily tasks with "unseeing" eyes, but just imagine how much richer and more fulfilling our lives would be if we noticed everything that we could see. True relaxation comes from our full appreciation, through all the faculties available to us, of the world around us, good or bad.

One of the most wonderful things about sight is its ability to discern shade and colour. Each colour vibrates at its own "light frequency" and can have a profound effect on our vitality, emotions and well-being. Shades of blue and violet are restful, lowering blood pressure and decreasing pain, but they can also cause depression if we wear blue when feeling low. Energizing red light fills us with vitality, but can also cause stress levels and blood pressure to rise if we are already angry or agitated. Pale pink calms us, and may even relieve headaches – it was found that migraine sufferers have fewer attacks when wearing rose-tinted spectacles. Yellow stimulates our intellect, but may also cause insomnia or nervous tension. Cool green is calming – it reduces anxiety and helps us to recover after an illness.

Exercise 7
Hues of Relaxation

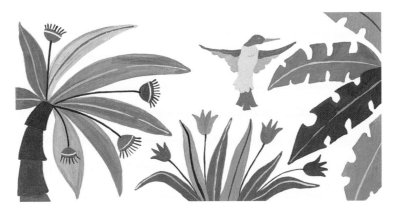

Using our imagination to visualize a peaceful place, filled with a variety of rich and vibrant colours, will help us to relax. We can also recover from troubles and ills by drawing upon the healing powers of colour.

• Find a quiet time and lie down on your bed or a comfortable couch. Close your eyes. Use your imagination to retreat to a secret garden. It is safe and warm, and filled with lush, tropical foliage in all the shades of green you can imagine. Here and there you can see glimpses of other colours, in the form of vibrant blue, yellow, orange and red flowers.

• Imagine an emerald green humming-bird hovering in the air above you. Notice the golden dappled sunlight filtering down between the leaves of exotic palms and giant ferns. You can just glimpse a clear blue sky. The scents of vanilla, orange and jasmine fill the air.

• Explore all the sights of your tropical garden as much as possible. Let yourself drift deeper into a relaxed, meditative state. When you have finished, reassure yourself that you can always return to this tranquil place, simply by closing your eyes and conjuring it up in your mind.

Scent and Aromatherapy

Think back to the scents of childhood – the rich, comforting aroma of a favourite chocolate cake, the smell of freshly cut grass in a sunny summer garden, the comforting menthol ointment that soothed away our coughs and colds. We are instantly transported back to a secure, carefree and happy time. Our sense of smell has an amazing evocative power. This is because it is linked directly to the part of the brain that governs our memories, instincts and emotions.

We can use scent, and its powers of association, to improve our well-being and keep us stimulated and energized, or calm and relaxed, during the most challenging of times. One of the most popular remedial and preventative therapies is aromatherapy. Essential oils, extracted in minute amounts from aromatic plants and herbs, have been used for thousands of years to cure ills, both mental and physical – ancient Chinese and Persian texts mention them, and Hippocrates, the Greek father of medicine, recommended scented oils for relaxation.

Although many essential oils are now readily available from specialist shops, the relaxing properties of scents need not be bottled to work their magic on our well-being. Next time you are outdoors, try to distinguish as many scents as you can. You may be surprised at the richness and variety of scents that surround you every day. Think about your favourite smells – they may be coffee, herbs used in cooking, or the sweet smell of roses. During times of stress, surrounding yourself with them will help you to relax. Using an oil burner will enable you to bring any scent you like into your home. But instead of buying store-made oils, place a few petals or leaves of your favourite flower or herb together with a couple of teaspoons of water in the burner. Light the candle inside the burner, and, as the temperature of the water rises, the delicious scent will flood the room.

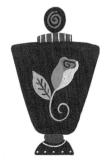

Exercise 8
Aromatic Bathing

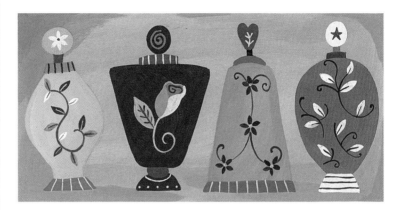

You can do the following exercise in a bath scented with ten drops of your chosen essential oil diluted in two teaspoons of carrier oil, or alternatively by using an essential oil burner in a scent-based meditation. (Important: if you are pregnant or ill, always consult a doctor before using any essential oils.)

• Choose an essential oil that appeals to you – for example, ginger is an aphrodisiac, peppermint is invigorating, lime will raise your spirits and violet or lavender will help you to relax.

• Sit or lie comfortably and close your eyes (if you are in the bath, make sure that the water is not too hot). Take five deep breaths – taking care to breathe from your abdomen and not your chest. Allow the scent of your chosen essential oil to fill your entire body. Imagine it coursing through your veins, invigorating and yet relaxing every part of you.

• Slow your breathing to a gentle rhythm, and try to still your thoughts so that you experience the scent alone. Meditate like this for around fifteen minutes and then open your eyes and very slowly and gently stand up. You feel refreshed and calm.

A Matter of Taste

We all too often overlook the importance of taste even though it plays a huge part in our daily lives. Think about your favourite food. Why is it your favourite? Does it hold happy memories for you? Is your mouth beginning to water as you think about it? Taste, like smell, has many powerful associations with the past.

Appreciating taste can be a wonderfully sensuous way to relax. In some countries, such as those of the Mediterranean, leisurely meals form the cornerstone of traditional family life. They often continue for several hours and many generations sit down together. Taking our time to eat allows the calming benefits of taste to reveal themselves. If we eat quickly we don't appreciate the tastes as well as we could. The next time you sit down to eat, consciously try to slow down the meal. As you chew, try to discern each separate taste in the food. Notice how the flavour of the food changes as you chew it and feel its texture on your tongue. Consider how each taste complements the other flavours in the meal. As you eat, mindful of your food, you are bound to feel more relaxed. Eating this way is also healthier – we are less likely to overeat and more likely to chew our food properly, thus helping our digestion and reducing the likelihood of heartburn.

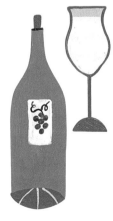

You may try to include an appreciation of taste as part of a relaxation exercise. Depending on the season, choose a fruit that you enjoy eating. Perhaps you'll try cherries in the spring, plums in the summer, apples in the autumn or oranges in the winter. Sit comfortably and relax your body. Drink some water to clear your palate, and then take a bite of your chosen fruit. Hold it in your mouth. Fix your entire attention on the taste sensation. You don't need to worry about anything, just enjoy this natural, wholesome food, abundant with health-giving properties.

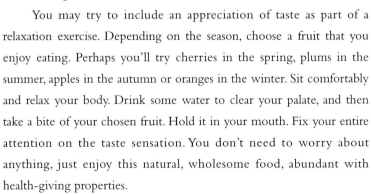

Exercise 9
A Dinnertime Relaxation

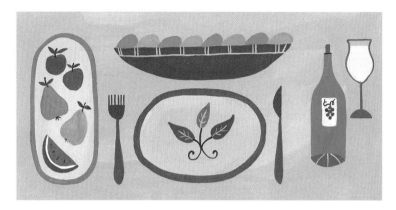

Set aside one night a week or month to enjoy a meal with family or friends. Take it in turns to cook, or each cook a course, and let the evening drift away in the relaxed company of people and tastes that you love.

• Ensure that when you and your family or friends eat, you can concentrate on the food and on each other. Choose a night when no one has to run off to a club, see friends or retire to the study to work.

• Create a welcoming and warming atmosphere by putting on some favourite soothing music, and lay the table attractively – perhaps place a vase of garden flowers on the table, or light some candles.

• When the food is brought out, take a few moments to allow all your senses to appreciate it. Look at the rich colours and smell the aromas drifting up from the plates. Say a few words of thanks to the cook.

• Make a point of not talking with your mouth full, nor hurriedly swallowing your food to join a conversation. This meal can take as long as any of you needs to really enjoy every last mouthful and each other.

Quality Rest

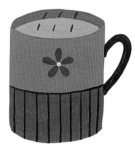

Bring to mind the feelings of waking slowly from a blissful, peaceful sleep. Our limbs feel totally relaxed and heavy, the bedclothes are draped snugly around us, and the bed feels firm beneath us, yet accommodating to the contours of our body. We ease ourselves into consciousness, notice the morning sun streaming in through the window, and anticipate the smells and tastes of our breakfast. We lie for a few moments and enjoy these feelings of relaxation. If we could wake up like this each morning, relaxation would be our companion from the very start of the day.

Quality sleep is essential for the well-being of our mind, body and spirit. It is a period of profound rest during which our muscles relax, and our bodies can rejuvenate and repair themselves after a day's wear and tear; our minds can sort out the vast amounts of information which flood our brains during the day; and our dreams help us to make sense of problems and issues that face us. But, paradoxically, if we are over-tired or over-anxious, sleep may elude us. Our resulting tiredness makes it harder for us to deal with the next day's activities and we find it more difficult to deal with stress. As a result, we become more anxious and our sleeplessness just seems to get worse. This is why it is so important to wind down and relax at the end of the day (see box, right).

The amount of sleep we need varies for each individual. In general, however, the younger we are, the more sleep we naturally receive. As babies we spend fourteen to sixteen hours asleep every day; as five year olds we sleep for an average of twelve hours; most adults get by on seven to eight hours; and, for the elderly, five or six hours a night is sufficient. If you have been ill, or have endured a long period of stress, try to find the time for extra sleep. You will allow your body to rejuvenate and recover properly, ready for your next challenge.

Strategies for a Good Night's Sleep

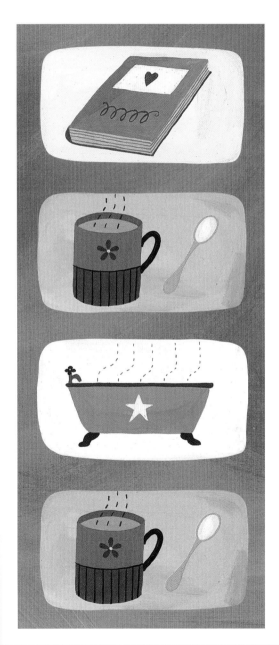

Unfortunately, when we are stressed sleep is one of the first things to suffer, even though we need its restorative powers more than ever.

Try to go to bed at a regular time each night and get up at the same time in the morning. Make sure your bed is comfortable, and your bedroom is dark, quiet and warm. Try to avoid napping during the day, because you will find it harder to sleep later.

Regular exercise can help you sleep, but don't do anything too strenuous late in the evening. Too much food, caffeine, nicotine or alcohol late at night will also disrupt your sleep (alcohol may help you drop off, but you will have a disturbed night once its effects have worn off).

Before you go to bed, take some time to unwind from the stresses of the day – listen to some soothing music or luxuriate in a candle-lit bath. A warm drink may help you relax – hot milk with cinnamon or nutmeg or a herbal tea for example.

If you can't sleep, get up and leave the room. If you have something on your mind, write it down and promise yourself you will deal with it in the morning. Spend a few minutes taking deep breaths and clearing your mind, then go back to bed and try to fall asleep once again.

The World of Dreams

Dream sleep

We move through cycles of sleep every night. Initially, we sleep lightly and then move into a deeper and more profound sleep. After about ninety minutes, we rise into what is known as rapid eye movement (REM) sleep. It is during this stage that we dream. In REM sleep our brain activity levels rise, blood-flow to the brain increases, and we twitch our eyes rapidly beneath the lids. Toward the beginning of the night, our periods of REM sleep may last only about fifteen minutes out of every ninety, but as the night wears on, our dream sleep increases to half an hour. If we are woken during REM sleep, we are very likely to remember our dreams.

We all dream, every night, even though we may not always remember our dreams when we wake. The mysteries of why we dream are far from solved, but dream experts agree that dreams act as a safety valve. Using symbols, dreams allow us to work through our emotions, thoughts and anxieties so that we can start afresh each day. Taking note of our dreams, and using their images and symbols to help us solve problems, can offer a unique guide to matters of waking life. In the words of the Jewish *Talmud*: "A dream that is not understood is like a letter which is not opened."

Many ancient cultures believe that our dreams represent a profound communication between our souls and the spirit world. Dreams are seen as opportunities to learn from the wisdom of a wider consciousness. In parts of Africa, the Americas and Siberia, shamans or witchdoctors find spiritual guidance in their dreams to cure people from mental and physical diseases. Ancient Greeks, such as Hippocrates and the philosopher Aristotle, believed that dreams could be used to diagnose and treat illness. In other traditions, such as those of the Middle and Far East, dreams are regarded as instruments to bring insights, prophecies and warnings to our attention.

More recently, psychoanalysts Sigmund Freud and Carl Jung regarded dreams as unique windows into our state of mind. Freud believed that our dreams contain symbols of our repressed desires. Even if the meaning of a dream remained unclear, according to Freud the act of dreaming itself expresses these hidden emotions and helps to heal our psyche. Freudian dream analysis uses a process called "free association". To try this, write down the first thing that comes to mind after thinking of your dream. Continue listing any associations until you have twenty or so. See if your list reveals anything to you. For

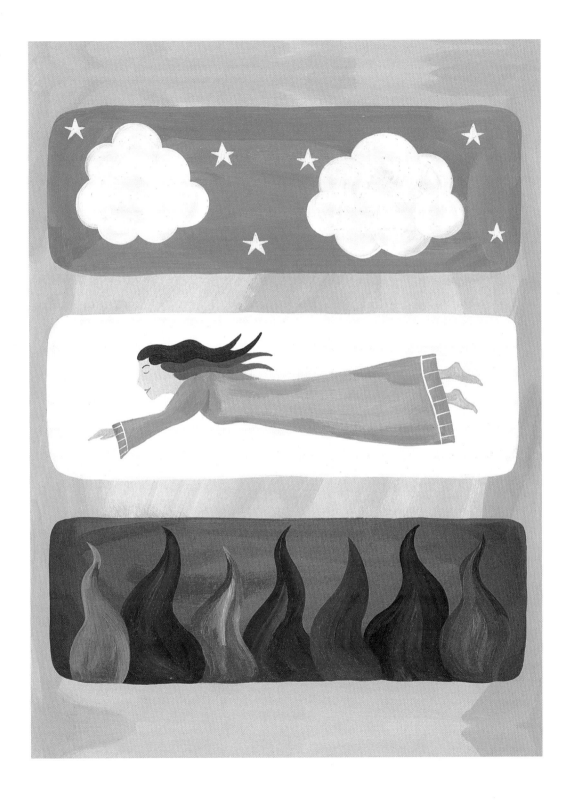

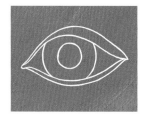

example, "maze, wall, door, lock, and so on" may reveal a theme of being trapped – perhaps deep down you wish to find a new career, or are unhappy in your relationship.

Jung, on the other hand, used a method he called "direct association" to interpret dreams. Write down your central dream image in the middle of a piece of paper – for example, the vision of you falling from a great height or flying through the air. Circle this central image and around this circle write down all the images and comments that seem intuitively appropriate. You may realize that the idea of falling echoes the feelings of powerlessness you feel at work, or you may feel that you don't have enough emotional support in your life. When you have finished, consider the combination of all your associations and the dream image to arrive at an interpretation.

When we fall asleep we expect to be able to relax and escape from the problems of the day. But sometimes our nights are filled with busy, vivid, thought-provoking and even unsettling dreams. In times of trouble we may find our dreams are disturbing or frightening, and we wake feeling anxious and tense. Investigating the root of this type of dream is essential for our relaxation. Nightmares – which are dreams accompanied by a feeling of horror or distress – may indicate a serious problem or fear that we need to address. In nightmares deep-seated emotions of frustration, repression or self-condemnation invade our thoughts and interrupt our peace. However painful it seems, we should try to bring these negative emotions to the surface. During the day write or draw the subject of your nightmare on a piece of paper. Does it seem obvious to you what it represents? Think about ways in which it may relate to your life. For example, if, in your dream, you were chased by a murderer wielding an axe, are you feeling hounded or threatened by someone in real life? Think about ways in which you can improve the situation. Even if there is no way to do this, simply working out the possible meaning of your nightmare will help you to feel calmer.

Sometimes nightmares can be so violent that we dread going to sleep the next night. Just before you retire for the night, try visualizing a pleasant, relaxing scene – such as a woodland during the autumn. Look at the coloured leaves on the trees, feel the slight sharpness and chill of the air on your face, and hear the crunch of fallen leaves underfoot. When you are feeling totally relaxed and peaceful, go to bed. These positive images will find their way into your subconscious and, hopefully, give you a fulfilling night's sleep.

Recurring dreams, whether pleasant or distressing, often convey an important message, which, if we do not heed it, keeps reappearing until we take note. Set aside a few minutes during the day, and lie down and close your eyes. Consciously relax all your muscles and gently begin to explore your recurring dream. Imagine that you are walking through the scene as a passive observer. As an "outsider" can you see any meaning to the dream? Once you have explored your dream as closely as you can, gently rouse yourself and begin to write down all the possible interpretations that spring to your mind, however ridiculous they seem. You may be surprised at the level of your insight. If the recurring dream reappears, repeat the process until you have solved its mystery and the dream ceases.

Dream problem-solving

We are all familiar with the concept that we should sleep on a problem in order to solve it. Test your powers of dream problem-solving by asking a friend or partner to set you a puzzle (perhaps an anagram) to solve in your sleep. Visualize the puzzle, but do not seek to solve it, as you drift off – hand it over to your unconscious to work on during the night. When you wake up, you may find that the answer is revealed literally; if not, the resolution may appear in the form of a visual or verbal pun, couched in dream symbolism. Explore your dream and see if it has revealed the answer.

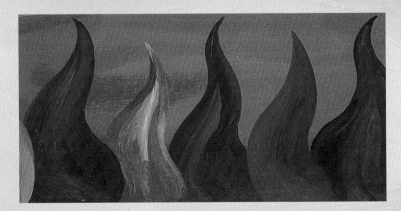

Summing Up

- Breathe deeply – renewed energy and peace will flood your body and mind.

- Meditate to clear your mind of worry. Just a few minutes a day will help you feel balanced and at peace.

- Stretch out the stress. Feel the tension flow out of your muscles and drift far from your thoughts.

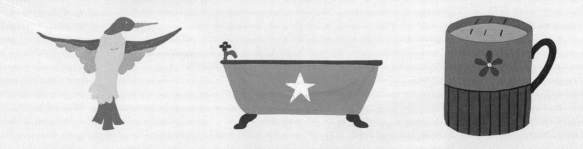

- Make a haven of calm. Surround yourself with beautiful objects and sounds, and delicious scents and tastes.

- Reach out and hug your partner, your children and your friends.

- Get the most out of sleep. Give your body time to recharge and your mind the chance to dream your worries away.

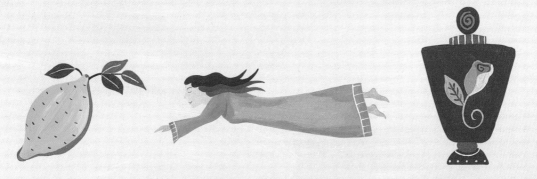

The Inner Realm

Our inner realm is the home of true relaxation and deep happiness. We can tap into its truthfulness by listening to the wisdom of our intuition and learning how to use our powers of reason. Knowing when to accept all that life deals us and when to take control, learning to change our attitudes and circumstances without fear of failure or responsibility, and discovering how to see the beauty and goodness in all things, will bring us closer to permitting the serene inner self to shine through whatever happens. In these ways the inner realm shows us how to be calm, confident and self-assured in all aspects of our lives.

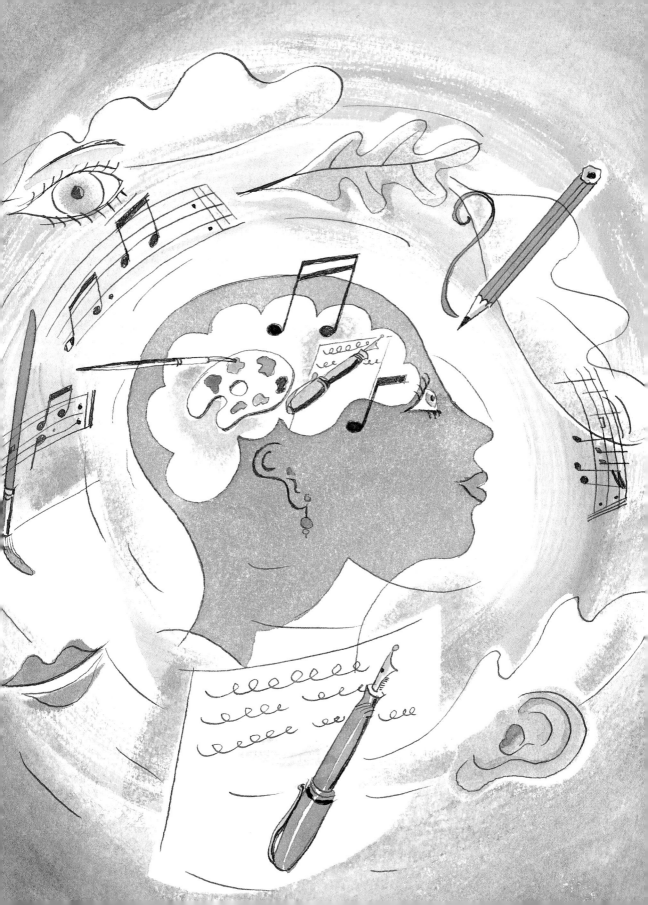

Instinct, Reason and Intuition

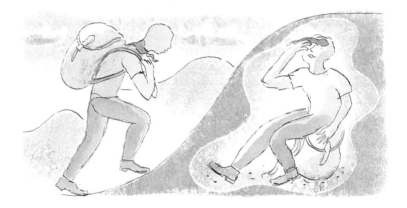

We have at our disposal three processes by which we can arrive at a decisive action or a plan. The most basic of these is instinct – an innate behavioural reaction to external stimuli that reminds us of our animalistic nature. Instinct usually follows a fixed pattern of behaviour which is predictable: for example, if we put our hand into boiling water, we will instinctively withdraw from the pain. Our instincts have ensured the survival of our species for thousands of years. However, they are automatic, so we have little control over the decisions that they make for us. We *can* overrule our instincts (we use this ability as a method of overcoming phobias: by halting the instinctive reaction to irrationally perceived danger we give ourselves time to see that no harm can come to us), but it takes effort. A more relaxed attitude is to remember that our instincts are there to keep us safe and to let them do their job.

Reason, the second decision-maker, is the power of the mind to think, understand and form judgments by a process of logic. When you bought this book, you thought about its contents; you understood that they are intended to help you relax through easily understood techniques; and you judged that the book would fulfil its purpose and that you would find it useful – you deemed it logical to buy the book. Often such reasoning happens in an instant and we do not register the mental rationalizing that leads us to take a particular course of action. Nevertheless reason is the process by which most of our decisions are made and it is entirely in the realm of our control.

Understanding reason is a valuable key to beating stress. If we are unsure about a decision, we feel anxious. Although it would be impossible to eradicate all traces of uncertainty in decision-making, we can reduce the risks. Make an effort to break down each of your reasoned decisions into its components: thought, understanding and judgment. A stressful decision is made when we skip from thought to judgment, thus defying logic. Say we decide to buy a car: if we have the thought, make the judgment and go ahead and buy the car without understanding what it means to us to do so, we subsequently have to deal with an often angry internal monologue that can't understand why we thought about buying the car in the first place. Rationalizing after the event is stressful, because the event itself cannot be changed.

Of course, this doesn't take into account our third decision-making power – intuition. This is the ability to understand something without the need for conscious reasoning – it is an innate sense of when something is right or wrong, good or bad. Our intuition will pick up on unconscious clues about a given situation. For example, we can often sense tension in a room full of people before we have any logical reason to suspect the truth. However, intuition can cause stress when we are not brave enough to trust in it. In the pursuit of logic, we often dismiss our intuition as trickery of the unconscious; we have taught ourselves to mistrust it, because it cannot be scientifically explained. In many respects, rectifying this requires blind faith: only by following the messages of our intuition, so that these messages prove themselves to be true, will we build up confidence in our internal radar. We should remind ourselves that, just as instinct keeps us safe from danger and reason permits us to perceive what is logical, intuition represents a profound, innately truthful, higher self that will always lead us along the best path if we have the courage to let it be our guide.

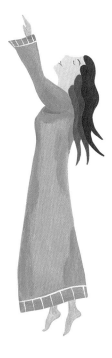

Acceptance versus Control

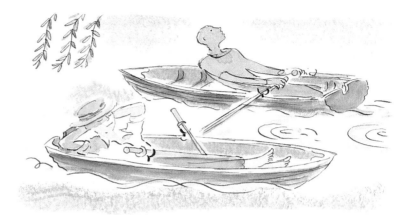

Think back over your day. Were you happy to go with the flow all day, or were there times when you felt like resisting – when you wanted to put the oars back in the rowlocks and row yourself and others hard in your own direction? The opposing forces of acceptance and control play a significant part in the way we manage our lives and also have a fundamental impact on how relaxed we feel, day to day.

We might tell ourselves that if we accept all that life throws at us, without question, then we begin to live a passive life that wanders a somewhat aimless path along an empty road. Nothing is further from the truth. Perhaps a better way to view acceptance is as "a willingness". If we accept a gift from someone, we have shown a willingness to receive that gift; if we accept all that life presents us with, we have shown a willingness to face the realities of our existence, move or work through them and come out richer on the other side. In this respect, acceptance becomes less of a synonym for passive non-reaction and more of a vehicle for displaying strength of character. What is crucial, if we are to succeed at showing willingness, is that we have total self-acceptance. We should strive to be confident about who we are and what we want to achieve, so that no matter what hurts or upsets us on the outside, we are certain that on the inside, in our inner realm, we are good, pure, peaceful, truthful and strong, and able to cope with anything with an attitude of complete calm.

In order to live a relaxed life we must establish what things we can and cannot control. The principles are simple – in fact, there is only one principle to follow: the only things over which we have control are the actions of the self. In practice this is a surprisingly difficult principle by which to live. Have another think about your day. Try to recall all your interactions with others in as much detail as possible – how many people did you try to persuade to do something that you wanted them to do, against their own natural instinct? Perhaps you tried to persuade a colleague to tackle a project in your way, or perhaps you simply positioned your hand when receiving change so that the shop assistant had to give you your money in a certain fashion – say, notes between your thumb and finger and coins in your palm. Exerting control over people can be as blatant or as subtle as you like. But now think about how you would have felt if your colleague had refused to undertake the project your way, or if the shop assistant had put the the coins on top of the notes, all into the palm of your hand. By trying to control something or someone, we make ourselves prey to frustration and anger should things not go our way – and we also exert unnecessary effort. Nature will bring to us all that is rightfully ours in due course.

The ancient Chinese Daoist principle of *wu wei* (literally meaning "non-action") works on the understanding that yielding to others, or to inevitable circumstances, is the most effective response to the problems of human existence. Action is believed to be created through inaction, as long as we do not oppose life's natural flow, and in this way all things can be accomplished. For example, a Daoist will not argue with another person. It is believed that there is a right and proper time for expressing the truth (each of us has our own individual truth – life-course – which we must follow). If the case for the truth is made at the wrong time (against nature) then conflict will ensue; if it is made at the right time (with nature) then it will be accepted amicably.

Working with, not against, the grain

Fighting for control is exhausting and often unsuccessful. If you often say to yourself: "I never make mistakes"; "I am always on time"; "I never show my emotions"; "I never delegate to others"; "I never deviate from the path I have set", you are probably making life harder on yourself than it need be. Strive toward a more relaxed acceptance of life. Phrases such as "I sometimes get it wrong"; "If I don't finish the job today, tomorrow will be OK"; "I am happy to achieve an outcome in its own time"; "I am not afraid of the future – life is an adventure"; "Freedom from anxiety is a goal in itself" are an indication of openness to the natural flow of nature, making for a wholly relaxed life.

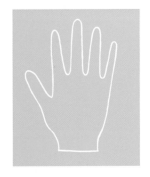

Making Changes

The Book of Changes

The ancient I Ching, *or Chinese* Book of Changes *(1000BCE) divines the likely outcome of any of life's changes. In the* I Ching, *64 hexagrams describe the effects of all of life's transitions, including conflict, ambition, exhaustion, relaxation and abundance. Coins or sticks are thrown in the air, and the pattern they make when they land is matched with one of the hexagrams. A solution can then be divined. If you are finding it hard to make a decision, try creating your own method of* I Ching *— throw up some coins. Is there a message in the way they have landed?*

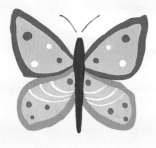

Change is inevitable and, if we are to be relaxed, we must be prepared to change. According to its dictionary definition, change is "an act or an instance of becoming different". Spend a few moments contemplating this explanation. When we feel stressed being "different" seems the thing farthest from our minds. We think that being or making things different will lead to more stress: making changes breaks the established pattern of our existence and we have to walk unchartered territory (see p.76). But if we feel discontented or frustrated in our present existence, why are we agitated by the prospect of changing ourselves (through our actions and attitudes) so that we don't feel those things any more? And it isn't just change of the self that unnerves us — all change is unnerving as it pushes us out of our comfort zones.

The first point to make is that feeling anxious over changing ourselves is a terrible waste of our precious, creative energy. The seat of our being — who we truly are — lies deep within, in our inner realm, and it cannot be influenced, battered or infected by anything. The core of our being is constant; but our attitudes toward, and feelings about, ourselves and our circumstances are not. We should never feel anxiety when faced with changing our attitudes or feelings: their nature is supposed to be one of transition and transformation. Rigidly sticking to what we think or feel about anything can only in itself breed stress. To live a relaxed life, we need to be able to go with the flow.

We fear changing our circumstances because intimately bound up in doing so is a sense of responsibility. If we set in motion change, then we are accountable for its consequences (but, as we will see, small changes can be effective, and they are much less worrying). So, we put up barriers to change, the most common one being "I don't have the time." This attitude exposes a fundamental misconception in the way

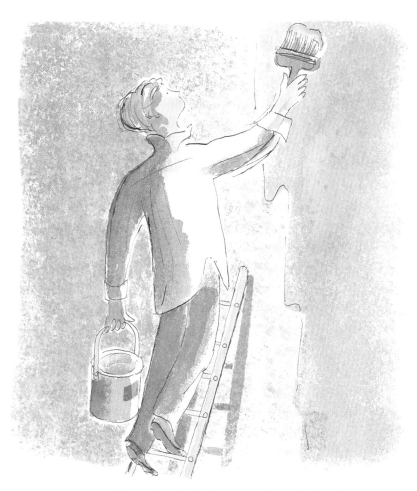

we view change. Most of us think that change has to be "big" or hugely time-consuming to make a difference. Instead of spending an hour clearing out a cupboard and throwing away the hoards of our accumulated chattels (many of which are often completely dispensable – without even being ruthless), we think that we have to move house in order to have more space. Instead of spending a day at the weekend doing nothing but our favourite pastime with our partner, say taking a long walk together in a beautiful area of countryside, we think we have to go on a vacation so that we can relax with the person whom we love. Of course, there are times when moving house or taking a vacation is needed, but usually change need not be time-consuming or difficult: small differences can have a big effect on our well-being.

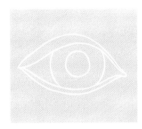

Think how refreshed you feel when you open a cupboard door and the items inside are stacked neatly with space to spare, rather than everything tumbling out on top of you. When reasoned logically (see pp.60–61), we see that there is nothing to fear from small but effective changes at all – most of which can be changed back if we are not happy with the outcomes they bring.

When it comes to long-term change (for example, making fundamental alterations to a relationship because it has gone sour), it helps to counter any fear by learning to view the ultimate change (say, making a new life on our own) as an attainable outcome reached by small, regularly placed stepping-stones of change ("goals"). This way we remove the fear that goes hand in hand with making an enormous leap of faith. Even if we have the self-confidence to make that leap without fear, once we have jumped many of us become unnerved by any potential consequences, and by our responsibility for them. We may sabotage the new course in order to return to the safety of our old circumstances – even if we hurt ourselves in the process. The exercise opposite will help you to set yourself stepping stones to change, gradually increasing your self-confidence so that you no longer fear the responsibility of the changes that you put in motion.

Whatever changes we make, one of the most important things to remember is that rather than viewing change as a source of stress, we should see it as an effective way of conquering stress. Actively changing our lives can be a cleansing, regenerative process, making space for renewed clarity to help us become calmer, more relaxed people, able to view our lives dispassionately and with proper perspective. In addition we should always be reminded that, no matter what happens outside ourselves, our inner realm is constant and invulnerable to change.

Exercise 10
Setting Goals

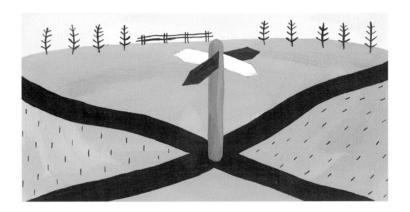

Setting short, attainable goals helps us to establish a clearly defined purpose toward long-term positive change. Use this exercise to practise goal-setting.

• What would you like to achieve in different areas of your life after, say, one year? Find goals for the categories of family, work, health, relationships, personal development and leisure.

• Write down your goals and devise five steps to help take you to each one. If necessary, talk to a friend (who will have an uninvolved clarity) to help you keep your aims in perspective. One by one, visualize yourself achieving your goals. This will help to increase your motivation and help you to see how your aims can come within your grasp.

• Work out plans to take you to the first goal in each category. When you actually attain each one, give yourself a reward. Repeat the process for the next set, and so on. If you find yourself unable to reach a goal, don't feel disappointed – think imaginatively about how you might modify your goals to achieve them. Are you being unrealistic? Do you need to create more stepping-stones to get where you want to go?

Developing Perspective

Bird's eye view

As you sit at home, mulling over a problem, imagine stepping outside your body and floating up above yourself. In your mind's eye notice the room you are in. Move your point of vision beyond the room and observe the surrounding garden; see your neighbours and your street. You are now flying in the sky. Your house is one of many below you. Fly higher and see the town nestled in the countryside. Keep moving away until you are far into space: the world, and within it your problems, is a tiny speck among thousands of undiscovered and wonderful planets. Do your concerns seem so vital now?

When anxiety builds up we lose our sense of perspective, so that minor irritations begin to take on outsized proportions. Without perspective we compound stress, because the more burdened we feel the more the relative importance of things becomes distorted.

Spend a few moments now thinking about a recent time when you snapped at a loved one because of an innocent or minor mistake they had made – perhaps your father had not put the telephone receiver back on the hook properly and you had been trying to call them. Although they may be irritating, such occurrences, viewed dispassionately in the context of our whole lives, often do not warrant the explosive reactions that we give them.

Before we can begin to regain our perspective, it is good to understand that the inflated importance we place on minor irritations is a symptom of our stress, not its cause. And the telephone being off the hook, say, acts as a trigger for the release of our otherwise pent-up anxiety. With these realizations, we can look for the true cause of our stress and start to develop some proper perspective.

When a friend experiences a crisis we often find that we are able to see a solution that our friend cannot: while they are emotionally caught up in the problem, we are separate from it. Hearing the views of a detached listener on your own problems is one way of developing perspective. However, if we prefer not to impose too heavily on our friends, we have to become a friend to ourselves. Taking your problems in turn, write down the bare facts on a piece of paper – use no adjectives or emphasis. With only the hard evidence before you, how important does each dilemma seem? How would you advise a friend who came to you with any of these things as a stressful concern? Prioritize the problems on your list and begin to deal with them, one by one.

Emptying Bottles of Stress

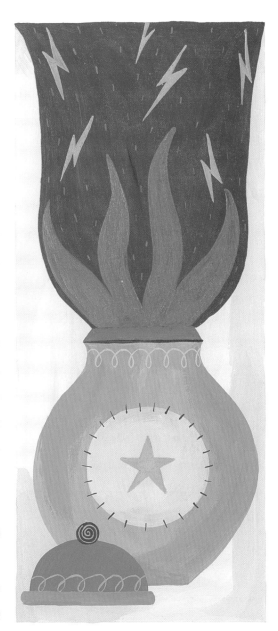

Most of our stresses build up little by little – a worry about one of our children adds to a niggle with our partner and concerns about a meeting at work, and before we know it, we are feeling overwhelmed. Out of embarrassment or habit, most of us internalize our thoughts, even when problems become burdensome.

Yet, bottling things up is one of the worst things we can do in times of stress. If our problems are always there, locked away inside us, consciously or unconsciously they will bubble away, until eventually, they explode out of the internal "bottles", often damaging our health or emotional well-being as they do so.

From time to time make a conscious decision to open your "bottles" of stress. As you release each issue in your mind, you will find it much easier to step back and view it rationally. Externalizing permits us to develop new and constructive perspectives on our concerns. Once each bottle is open, the problem inside is set free and is easier to resolve. If you find it hard to identify your problems, keeping a diary or finding a friend to ask you probing questions will help to clarify what issues you have stored away, so that you can look at them afresh and deal with them safely.

Hope and Disappointment

The wheel of fortune

The way disappointment and hope follow one from the other is perfectly embodied by the wheel of fortune. The disappointment of losing the lottery today is instantly replaced with the hope of winning tomorrow, as the wheel of fortune spins. The symbol of the wheel was used in medieval times to demonstrate the ups and downs of life, and that no matter what is destined to befall us, hope is sure to return.

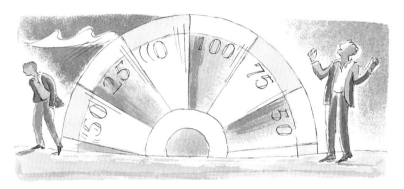

The disappointment we might feel at the death of the summer flowers in our garden rapidly turns into the hope of the growth of our autumn blooms; the disappointment we experience when an expected letter does not arrive, is soon followed by the hope that it will arrive in the mail tomorrow. Disappointment and hope are different sides of the same coin, they are mutually dependent and intimately joined – without one there cannot be the other. But it is important to make clear that disappointment and hope are not opposites – a sense of disappointment is not the same as a sense of hopelessness, just as feeling hope is not the same as feeling fulfilment.

For many of us hope seems difficult to sustain. We feel that if we permanently hope for the best we lay ourselves open to the possibility of continued disappointment. It seems easier on ourselves to expect disappointment – that way good things are lovely surprises and we can never feel let down. The trouble is that if we expect to be disappointed, disappointed is what we will be. Our attitude is such that no matter what good things befall us, we will perceive that they are not as good as they could have been. So, in order to live a relaxed life we need to spring-clean our attitudes – life's journey is filled with ups and downs, but these undulations make for a terrain that is unpredictable, exciting and full of positive experiences.

Make some time to sit down and divide your life into its major categories. These might be work, family, home, friends, and interests or hobbies. Give each category its own sheet of paper. Divide each sheet into three parts: "good points", "improvable points" and "aims". Taking each piece of paper in turn, make lists in the three parts, being as honest, thorough and specific as you can. Once you have completed each piece of paper, look at what you have put in the "improvable" section. Can any of these things be matched to what you have said in your "aims" box? For example, if you feel that your level of responsibility at work is "improvable", is there something in the "aims" box that would make the improvement? You may aim for more budgetary control or more staff to manage, or perhaps something more general, listing simply "a new job" within the next year. Try to make sure that each improvable point has a corresponding aim. Do this for each life category and review the results. What have you learned? Firstly, although there are improvements to be made in your current life (we might say that these are the areas that have disappointed you), there are also aims to pursue. Secondly, every part of your life has some good points – those good points (and your aims) are the champions of hope that will keep you strong during uphill stretches of life's road.

A warning, however: be realistic. A sense of permanent disappointment is often fuelled by hoping for too much. Although it is possible to reach almost any target we set, taking things slowly and building up a string of little hopes that have been fulfilled is, day to day, far more rewarding than setting ourselves one far-reaching target and then stumbling when we are only part way there.

Another good way of filling our life with hope is to try to see the positive in everything around us. Negative thinking saps our energy by internalizing our pain, meaning that hope seems something beyond our reach. Begin by distinguishing the positive experiences brought to you by your senses: the touch of your partner to reassure you; the chatter of people in the street reminding you of the comfort in communication between friends; and so on. Even if you can't feel or hear these things at the moment, conjure them up in your imagination. Then, what can you actually see before you? Perhaps the sunlight is reflected off glass; or a beautiful vase of flowers sits on the mantlepiece. Study in detail each object that you can see – it doesn't matter if the objects seem mundane – think about how each one uses space and contains space, and how each part of it works with others to form a three-dimensional whole. You might even see something that you do not like the look of – perhaps a plant has a dead leaf, or a cup has a chip in the rim. Imagine flowing all your recent disappointments into that one flaw and then focus on all the good before your eyes. The other leaves on the plant are lush, green and brimming with life; the cup is beautifully decorated and holds delicious and restorative tea for you to drink.

Also remember that hope in one area of our lives can feed into other areas. Positive thinking is contagious – once we see it making us happier in one aspect, it soon catches on in another! Developing and nurturing many supportive relationships with family, friends and colleagues will give us a positive base from which to fill other parts of our lives with hope. The family also provides a wonderfully safe environment in which to talk about our disappointments, let them go and move on. Taking regular physical and mental exercise (even if it is as simple as walking the dog, and doing a ten-minute meditation each day) will help us to feel more positive about our bodies and minds, which will soon feed into the way we feel about life generally – we will be filled with a new sense of confidence for ourselves and life.

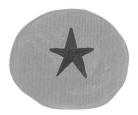

Most of all, remember that no matter what disappointments or frustrations befall us, hope is always there on the other side of the same coin: we just have to remember to flip the coin over to see it.

Exercise 11
Positive Commuting

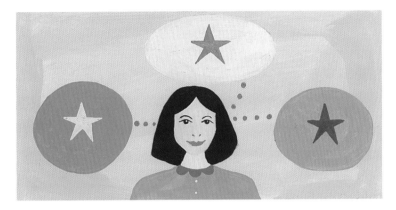

Changing our "self-talk" – the inner chattering of our minds – from negative to positive helps us to see the bright side of any situation. The following exercise uses commuting as its stressful situation – but you can adapt the method for any issue.

• Think of an occasion about which you habitually feel negative. It may be as you sit in your car, stuck in a traffic jam on your way to your office or workplace.

• As you imagine yourself in the car on the way to work, your familiar negative emotions come flooding back – the stress building up as you inch forward able to think only of the wasted time you are spending in the car. Out loud, say "lighten up!" to these negative thoughts.

• Consciously shift your negative attitude to a positive one. The slow progress of your journey gives you time for contemplation. Mentally organize your day so that when you arrive you are clearly focused.

• Practise this technique each time you travel to work – soon it will become second nature. Translate the system to other areas of your life.

Summing Up

- Trust in the wisdom of your intuition and the power of your reason to guide you along life's journey.

- Don't fight against your life. Bend with its twists and turns and you will find a path through any difficulty.

- Set yourself clear but flexible goals. You never know what's on the horizon.

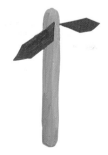 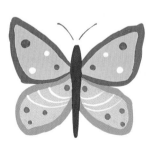 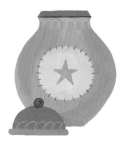

- Be confident in your decisions — if it feels right, it *is* right.

- Give yourself some distance from your problems. Look at things from more than one point of view.

- Keep alive your hope. Just as night follows day, fulfilment is bound to emerge from disappointment.

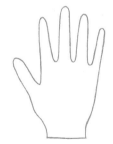 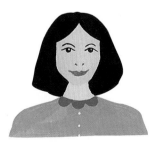 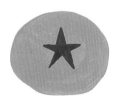

Expanding Your Horizons

For many of us relaxation means remaining within our "comfort zones" – routines, places and states of mind that seem reassuringly familiar to us, even if they do not provide us with peace. We tell ourselves that what lies beyond our familiar territories might be frightening or strange – better to stay where we are. However, true relaxation comes not from imprisoning ourselves in limited mental and physical space, it comes from expanding our lives, striding out beyond the "normal" and "habitual" to find inspiration and wonder in the far beyond. The world, with its revolving seasons and ever-changing terrain, is a wonderful and exciting place in which we can (and should) be free.

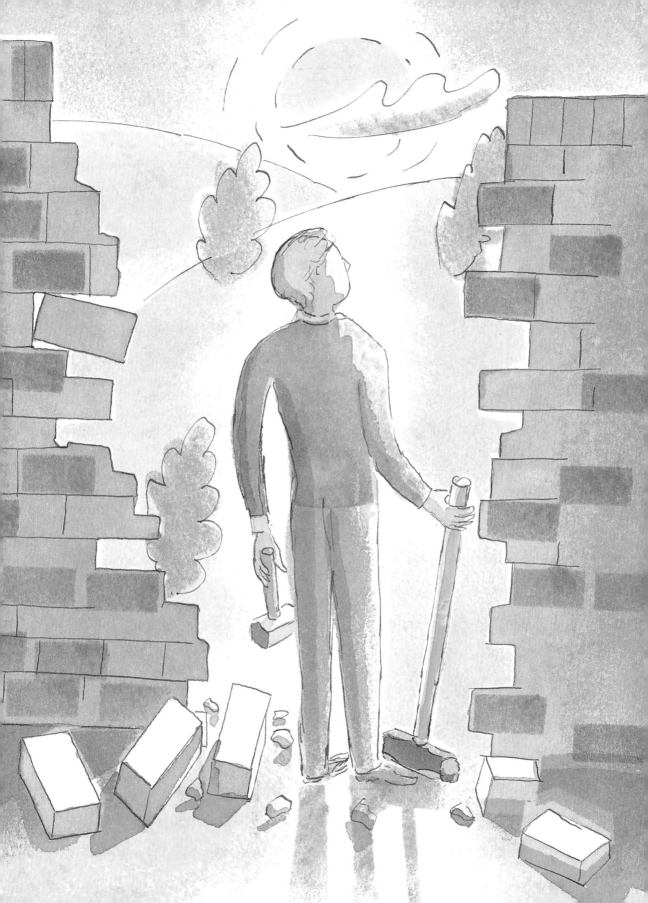

Freeing Ourselves from the Past

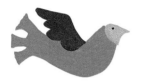

Birds of sorrow

When we are unable to let go of the past, painful events and memories may cast a shadow over the present. Sorrow and regret are common emotions, but, as an ancient Chinese proverb teaches, while we cannot prevent the birds of sadness flying over our heads, we can prevent them from nesting in our hair.

Our future may seem uncertain, and we may feel anxious about the present. The one thing that never changes is the past, and so for some it represents the ultimate security – a set of definites. It can be tempting during difficult times to focus on how things used to be. However, if we obstinately remain within the boundaries of that so-called security, the quality of each moment in the present is enjoyed only as part of the past. In order to relax we need to set ourselves free from our history.

Imagine that your past is a vast, dark cellar, hidden from the world by a heavy wooden door and secure lock. You step inside – it is cool and dry. Around the walls are rows of chests and jars. Each contains the treasures of your memories. Begin to explore the cellar. Open the jars one by one and let some memories flood out. You may remember a summer outing at which you made some new and wonderful friends; the time when you left home to start a new life in another city; or the moment when you were first introduced to your partner. Some memories are sad or uncomfortable, such as when you failed an examination or ended a relationship, but think about how you learned from your disappointments. And be proud as you rediscover your achievements. How do they affect your life now? Are there any lessons you wish to take with you from the cellar? Now look carefully at the cellar itself. It is dark, full of cobwebs, and dusty – it is not at all a healthy place to be. It holds all the experiences that have shaped you over time, but there is nothing friendly, warm or inviting about it. Now that you have spent some time there, you feel chilly. When you are ready, prepare to leave the cellar. Lock the door behind you and imagine stretching up on tiptoes to hang the key on a high hook. Your memories will always be accessible, but they reside in a place in which you would rather not live and they are not free to affect the present.

Exercise 12
Melting the Ice Sculpture

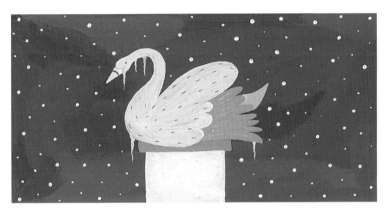

We may find it hard to let go of the past – especially if what lies ahead promises to be challenging. But the benefits of the present and future far outweigh the cost of leaving behind the past. This exercise will help you to move on.

• Close your eyes and imagine that you are walking through a frozen wilderness. In your path is a block of ice, representing your past. It is frozen in the shape of a beautiful bird, such as a swan.

• Think about your past difficulties. How are they affecting you now? For example, are you afraid to ask for a pay rise because you were refused one last time you asked? Mentally list the achievements you have made that would justify a higher salary. Praise your worth.

• As each positive thought enters your mind, it channels a gust of warm air onto the ice. The bird begins to melt, forming a pool of clear water.

• The pool represents your present. It is formed from the accumulated wisdom, knowledge, experience and actions of the past, but it is fluid – ever-changing and able to move itself around any obstacle.

Living for the Moment

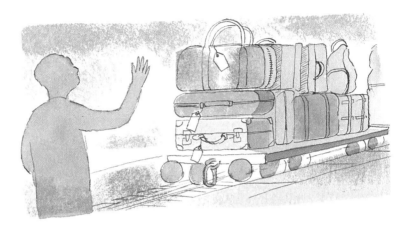

A wise person knows how to enjoy the moment. This is one of the most valuable and yet least-practised skills in our hectic, goal-driven society. Just for a minute close your eyes. Imagine casting off a weight from your back – roll your shoulders backward and feel the release of tension. Now imagine that all that you see before you is stillness (you might picture it as a calm pool of water, or a beautiful meadow with still grass on a windless day). There is total quiet – this is the perfect vision of the future. Allow the image to fade until you see nothing: the future is so calm that it needn't worry you. Breathe deeply and focus only on letting out a long, slow exhalation. For the duration of the out-breath, you are free from the heavy burden of the past which you have cast off, released from concerns about the future, and imbued with the essential spirit of the present – your breath. You have just lived by the words of French writer Albert Camus: "Real generosity ... consists in giving all to what is present."

Living for the moment offers us freedom from the shackles of all that has been, but also from all that will be. However, unless we make a special effort to turn our attention fully to the present, many of us find it difficult to cut ourselves free. There can be valid reasons for this: we may have many demands upon us and so we undertake one task thinking about what we have to do next; or we may find ourselves wondering if we should have handled the task we did a minute ago in a different way. Relaxation comes from simplifying each moment. Think about the times you have read a passage in a book and found that at the end of the page you haven't remembered a thing that's been written because your mind was buzzing with other thoughts. If the information that our brain has to process had been simplified – if we had focused upon each sentence on the page as we read it – the meaning would have been clear immediately.

Eastern cultures have much to teach us about appreciating just "being". For example, the Oriental philosophy of Zen Buddhism teaches its followers to apply the principle of "mindfulness" – keeping the mind fully absorbed in the task we are performing at any one moment, and literally meditating upon our actions and thoughts. Mindfulness is broken down into an awareness of several components: the movements and sensations of the body; mental states, such as moods and emotions; and mental objects, such as our thoughts and observations. Cultivating mindfulness involves being able to draw the scattered focus of the mind together into one unified point in the present. It involves calm and steady concentration. In this way we can become fully conscious in the moment, directly experiencing life without impediments.

Practise being mindful the next time your perform a task that you would normally find laborious. Perhaps when you are washing the car, loading the dishwasher or sweeping the yard. Instead of thinking ahead to the fun things or other tasks you might be doing later, or daydreaming perhaps about a holiday (past or future), focus fully on the moment. Try not to judge what you are doing – for example, sweeping is not a mundane job, it is simply sweeping. Allow the rhythm of your actions to absorb your consciousness and focus on the information you are receiving from your senses; listen to the sounds of the brush against the ground, look at the leaves piling up as you sweep. Once you become fully absorbed in the moment, even the worst, most routine jobs take on a new meaning – they become the calm focus of your consciousness.

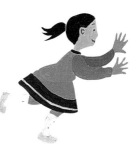

Trusting in the Future

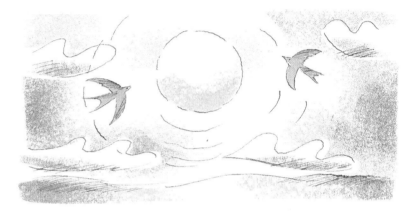

The future offers an intriguing mixture of mystery and apprehension. Friedrich Nietzsche, the 19th-century German philosopher, believed that "the present is influenced as much by the future as it is by the past". If we fear the future, we allow the darkness in the unknown to dim the light of our current lives. On the other hand, if we stop worrying about it, we can start to enjoy instead everything that we experience in the present.

We are all subject to the forces of change and destiny, and while we can make predictions based on instinct, reason, intuition and history, we can never be absolutely certain about what lies ahead. The pure fact of the matter is that we tend to fear what we feel we can't control. As we cannot control the passage of time, we make ourselves its victims, cowering at the mercy of the hand of fate. How many times have you found yourself asking "what if ...?": What if I become ill? What if my relationship breaks up? What if I lose my job? What if something happens to my child? But what if we stopped worrying about the what ifs? All the valuable energy used up in speculating about the future becomes free, ready for us to harness and enjoy in the present. Imagine yourself in your old age – how wonderful to be able to tell your grandchildren that one day you stopped worrying about the future and started to live each moment to the full.

This is not to say that we shouldn't do our best to make whatever lies ahead as easy on ourselves as possible. Remember that positive action today will resonate through time and bring positive reward tomorrow. Even if fate deals us a poor hand, positive thinking will make us feel strong, and we will be better equipped to cope with whatever befalls us.

If you have a specific fear of the future that looms in your mind, try to find a practical game-plan that will allay it. For example, if you are concerned about becoming ill, take active steps to try to maintain health by exercising regularly and eating well. If you are troubled about a relationship, open the channels of communication with your partner, and even seek relationship counselling as a preventative measure. The most effective way of overcoming a fear of the future is to have confidence in yourself – whatever happens, within you is the strength and resourcefulness to cope with it.

We should try not to dread the future, but neither should we create a fantasy of it in which all our problems have magically disappeared. Escapist thinking (in which we consistently focus only on a bright tomorrow) is common in people who are stressed. The fantasy is used as a way of avoiding the unpleasant reality of a difficult situation in the present – just as smokers or drinkers might increase their nicotine or alcohol intake as ways to relieve anxiety or blot out problems.

Instead of escaping into fantasy, face up to the problems of today. Think of this in practical terms. Today you feel anxious about a current problem. Unless you tackle that problem today it will still be there tomorrow and you will still feel anxious. Coping with adversity can result in valuable growth. It increases our confidence that we have the necessary inner resourcefulness to meet the challenges of the future. But there is little point in worrying about the future – we can't know the difficulties of what has not yet happened. All we can do is make the best preparations by living life to the full today – making good the problems of today, so that we can face tomorrow with a calm and happy heart.

Future visions

Visualization exercises may help if you feel apprehensive about the future or feel mired down in current problems. Sit in a quiet place where you feel safe and where you are unlikely to be disturbed. Take some deep, slow breaths to calm down and focus your mind. Now create a vision of the future as you want it to be. Picture yourself happy and successful in your job, harmonious in your relationships, healthy and energetic in yourself. Tell yourself that you deserve this future and that you have the ability to attain it. As soon as you start believing in yourself, you bring your hopes for the future within your grasp.

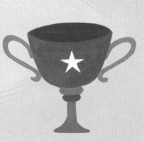

Nature's Balm

Imagine living each day like a flower: as the sun rises you gently tilt your head and open your petals to allow its all-giving energy to catalyze the biological processes essential for your survival; you gain nourishment from the natural world around you; and as the sun sets you draw in and rest. We might say that plants have the perfect existence – their very being governed by the rise and fall of the sun each day and the cycle of the seasons each year.

Humanity, however, is becoming increasingly estranged from natural cycles – and from nature itself. Artificial light gives sunrise and sunset minimal meaning to us; central heating and air conditioning mean that the cycle of the seasons have lost their immediate impact on our day-to-day lives. Most of us would shudder at the thought of returning to a state of natural surrender: if daylight hours were the only hours we could work, how would we find time to *do* everything?

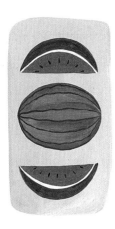

It would be impracticable to suggest that in order to shake off stress we need to retune our lives entirely to nature's rhythms. Neither do we need to pack up our city lives (70 per cent of people in the US live in cities; 60 per cent in the UK) and move to the countryside to benefit from the balming properties of nature. A small pot of flowers on a windowsill or a walk through a park can be enough to put us back in touch with the natural world, massaging our minds and lifting our spirits. Experience all the relaxing properties of a single flower. You might try meditating on the soft touch of its petals between your fingers; the gentle aroma that perfumes the air; or the pattern of its leaves. Meditate upon what the plant gives you: the cleanest, purest oxygen by which to breathe. In return you offer it the carbon dioxide essential for its survival. Every living thing is like an instrument in an orchestra, playing a harmonious balance of sound in nature's melody.

Exercise 13
Focus on Nature

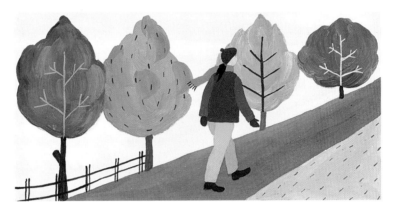

This exercise is intended to help sharpen your appreciation of nature and encourage your inner creativity. Try to repeat it in each of the different seasons, each time learning to reconnect with the natural world.

• Take a walk through your garden, in a park or in the countryside. As you walk focus fully on the air against your cheeks and the scents that it carries. Try to identify as many smells as you can. Now turn your attention to what you see. Notice the colours of the plants, trees, flowers, sky and clouds. Still looking, begin to open your ears to nature's sounds. Allow the melodies of birdsong, rustling leaves and trickling water to create a symphony in your consciousness. Touch all the leaves and flowers you can reach. Pay attention to their contours. How have all these sensations changed from previous seasons?

• Paying careful attention to any regulations in public places, collect leaves of as many different colours and shapes as you can. Even pick up blades of grass, fallen blossom, petals or twigs. When you return home, make a pattern or collage with the objects you have collected. Use this as a focus for meditation (see p. 35).

The Renewal of Life

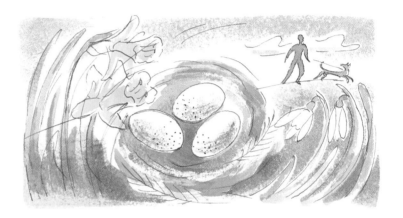

Spring is often emotionally linked with hopefulness. At this time we leave behind the long, dark nights of winter and look forward to the season of new life and promise. To attune yourself with the spirit of the season, spend a few extra moments lying in bed each spring morning and concentrate on the sounds you can hear – the tweeting of birds and the rustle of the wind through the new leaves on the trees.

As nature bursts forth with renewed energy, spring is a perfect time to review our lives and set in action positive, revitalizing changes. The tradition of spring-cleaning can be useful in heralding a new start. Clear clutter from your surroundings; open windows to allow fresh breezes to blow away the stale air of winter. As you sort through your home, imagine that the rooms represent areas of your life: the kitchen might correspond to your family; the bedroom your hobbies; and the study your work. As you clean each room, think of ways you can improve your quality of life in the corresponding area. Be as bold as you like: if you are getting married, paint your bedroom a harmonious colour, such as green; and perhaps plant a seedling to represent your new life – watch it grow as you move toward your shared goals.

Exercise 14
Absorbing the Energy of Spring

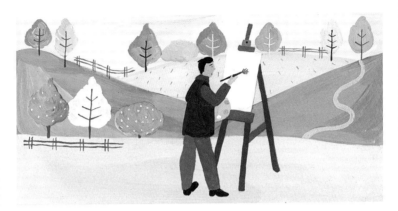

Prepare yourself for the changes of spring after winter, perhaps at the spring equinox (March 21 in the Northern hemisphere; September 21 in the Southern). Alternatively, this exercise can be used whenever you are feeling lethargic, burned out or uninspired and need to renew your energy and creativity.

• Lie on your back with your eyes closed and imagine that you are lying on the earth in a deserted forest. It is still winter. The ground feels cold, the air is harsh and the trees are bare.

• Imagine that as you lie there, the earth beneath you begins to warm up, until it feels like the spring sun on your back. On the trees young, lime-green shoots are unfurling their leaves. The air is alive with the scent of blossom and fresh grass. The brilliant yellow daffodils, and colourful crocuses and tulips, nod their heads in a refreshing breeze. Listen to the cheeping of chicks and the bleat of newborn lambs. All around you, there is new life.

• See yourself as part of this regeneration. The warmth that you feel is that of renewed energy. You feel refreshed and revitalized.

Summer and Freedom

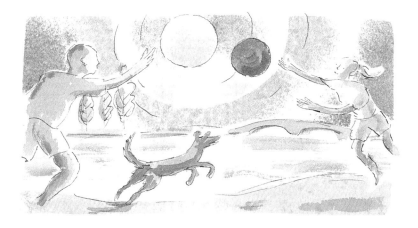

If spring is the season of birth, with budding leaves and flowers, then summer is the season of growth, when all the newness of spring blossoms into fullness and wisdom. Summer is traditionally a time of sunny days, long, light evenings and family vacations. In summer, time seems to grant us a wish and we feel that endless possibility is within our grasp. In Chinese philosophy, summer is symbolized by the Red Bird. It is the time of fire in which yang, the active energy, reaches its zenith, and yin, the passive energy, its nadir.

Summery moods are associated with plenitude, release and joyfulness. When we look around us we see abundance in the colours and scents of nature – flowers in full, colourful and aromatic bloom; trees which are full, lush and green; the ripples in water telling us that fish lie beneath in rivers and lakes. This is the season in which our problems seem to recede into the background. We should harness the sense of freedom that this gives, remember it and try to draw upon it even during our darkest hours. In summer, we can easily live to enjoy the moment – carry this with you at other times too.

Close your eyes for a moment and picture a seaside scene – it might be imaginary or real. Imagine that you can feel the warm sand underfoot as you walk along a deserted shore on a beautiful summer's day. Smell the salty air as your imaginary self looks at the water glistening in the light. Slow your breathing (see p.36) as you contemplate the regular ebbing and flowing of the waves. Imagine that each time a wave sweeps in, it brings with it a gift to help you to relax and deal positively with your challenges – it might be a token of love and support from a friend, a profound feeling of peace, a sense of better health after an illness or the whispering promise of spiritual riches.

Many of us maintain a strong emotional connection between summer and the lightheartedness of childhood. When we were young, the days during the long break from school seemed especially endless and were full of adventure. On a summer's day, try reconnecting with your childlike self and recapture your carefree attitude. Play outdoor games with your own children – splashing about in the water from a garden hose; if you live near the seaside, build a sandcastle on the beach – make it as elaborate as you can and then when you are done take a running jump into it, enjoying the exhilaration of this harmless destruction; go on a nature trail, looking at the beautiful patterned butterflies, the busy insects and the thickly leaved trees.

The midsummer solstice marks the longest day of the year (June 21 in the Northern hemisphere, December 21 in the Southern). In the West, ancient druids celebrated the solstice in a festival of light. Use this as inspiration to remind yourself of the abundance of the season and the benefits that the sunlight brings us. Have a celebratory party, and if possible entertain your guests outside. Decorate your garden or yard (or room, if you have your party inside) with lights. You might choose candles to represent the warming, energy-giving rays of the sun (be careful where you place these), and a garden lamp to represent the moon, which reflects the sun's light, reassuring us of the sun's continued presence even when it seems to have gone away. Little, white "fairy" lights (such as those used to decorate Christmas trees in the West) might represent the stars shining brightly through the darkness.

Sun power

The sun is the source of all energy in our solar system. It provides the earth with heat and light, without which life would be impossible. Many ancient peoples, such as the Aztecs, Incas and Egyptians, recognized the sun's vital power, and sun deities were central to their cultures and religions. Buy, or pick from your garden, some flowers (preferably sunflowers). When you get them home, think about how the sun's light enabled them to grow and bloom. What the sun does for these flowers, it can do for you, too.

Harvesting Life's Fruits

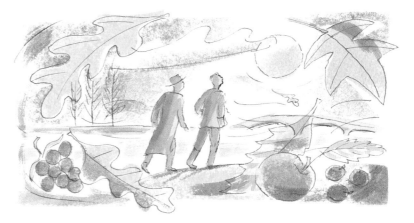

During autumn the promised abundance of summer is realized and crops are gathered to safeguard life during the coming winter. In many traditions autumn is a time of feasting, when fruits, vegetables and grains are blessed, and thanks are given for a good harvest.

Autumn states of mind are those of richness, generosity and abundance, when earlier toils have brought recognition, realization and success. This season symbolizes the calm and positive contemplation of what we have achieved, the skills and successes that we have accumulated over the previous months, and the storing-up of valuable experience for the future. It is a time when we may count our blessings, learning the value of what nature has given us, rather than coveting goods or striving for wealth or success. By appreciating the richness of your life you will feel more at peace and content as you prepare for winter.

To benefit from the spirit of autumn, whatever the time of year, take a moment to think about the good things in your life, and bring some happiness to other people. Tell your partner how important he or she is to you, or take your children on a special day out.

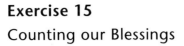

Exercise 15
Counting our Blessings

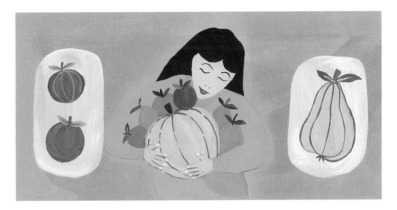

Much of the stress in our society comes from competition and striving for material success. It is all too easy to become caught up in this struggle which ultimately leads us to forget the most important and invaluable things in life. Try to take a few moments each day to count your blessings.

• Lie down in a quiet place and take some deep breaths to focus your thoughts. Close your eyes and turn your attention inward.

• Think carefully about your blessings. These may include good health, fresh air to breathe, water to quench your thirst and food to sate your hunger. You may have a loving partner, happy children, caring parents, supportive friends or an affectionate pet. You are free to enjoy the gifts of nature: the glory of a fall sunset or the colours of autumn leaves. Think about your skills, such as the ability to sing, cook a delicious meal or paint a picture, or your compassion for others.

• Now think of yourself as free from all the trappings of materialism – your bank account, your car. Without them you are at total peace, revelling in all that is good and true about life.

Retreat into Reflection

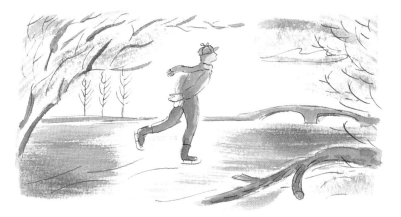

French writer Albert Camus once noted, "In the depths of winter, I suddenly learned that there was in me an invincible summer." An ability to find joy on the coldest nights and beauty in the most bleak and barren landscapes might indeed indicate that summer (or what it means to us) resides within. On a spiritual level, we might say the seasons are less to do with the weather, and more to do with our attitude to life. Take a few moments now to think of the things that you love about winter. Perhaps you enjoy the crisp, clear mornings; the incredible perfection in the symmetry of a snowflake; being the first to make footprints in fresh snow; the satisfying comfort of an open fire – or simply a warm home. Far from being a time of bleakness or misery, winter is a time of coming together (in the Northern hemisphere it includes the festivals of Thanksgiving, Christmas and New Year) and of the earth preparing itself for the new growth and life of spring.

Think about how and why animals hibernate, resting from the cold weather and restoring their energy to be bright, vibrant and full of vitality and purpose as soon as the warmer weather arrives. Think of winter as your own hibernation. In the long evenings, set about making a plan for the following year. In what ways do you hope that your home life will change? And your working life? What health goals do you want to achieve? Reflect on the past year and what it means for the future. Restore your energies with wholesome food and long periods of sleep – make sure that you get plenty of rest.

In Chinese philosophy, sluggish yin energy pervades during winter. But beneath the surface of all of us lies the vibrant yang, waiting to fill us with energy for the spring. Think of a frozen lake. On the surface the water is still and apparently lifeless, but beneath, the water continues to buzz with life – plants continue to grow and fish continue to swim, protected from the cold winter air by the icy topping on the lake. Beneath the frozen ground, seeds and bulbs lie ready to sprout into new life in the spring.

Winter is a time during which we need to be especially conscious of the warmth of human relationships. If you have an elderly neighbour or relative try to make a special effort to visit him or her more often. Perhaps give them a blanket or sweater to use on cold winter nights, or make them some soup, full of fresh, nutritious vegetables to warm and strengthen them. Ask if you can help with their shopping if it is difficult for them to walk on the icy sidewalks. At home bring together your friends and family. Eat wholesome, nourishing food together, play games and be sure to make lots of laughter. The next time you and your friends meet during winter, ask everyone to bring with them their favourite image of the season – a photograph of a beautiful winter memory, a fallen leaf, or bare twig. Encourage people to talk about what winter represents to them and what their goals are for the spring. Give each of your friends a small gift – perhaps a card with a collage of fallen leaves on the front. Inside, write a message of good will to encourage the spirit of human kindness and emotional warmth.

Most of all, feel heartened by the spirit of winter. For the Chinese, winter is symbolized by the Black Tortoise – an emblem of long life and indestructibility. No matter how cold or bleak the season seems to get, our spirits can never be frozen, and we can be assured that round the corner lies an invigorating spring.

Winter myths

One of the most famous myths about winter is the Greek tale of Persephone. She was the daughter of Demeter, the Goddess of fertility and the earth. Persephone was abducted by Hades, the God of the Underworld. Demeter's fury at the loss of her daughter caused her to put a blight on the land, threatening to starve humanity. Persephone was eventually rescued, but because she had eaten some of the food of the dead while she was in the underworld, it was decided that she must spend one-third of every year in Hades. This third of the year was winter, when Demeter made the land bleak and fruitless before renewing life with the return of her daughter in the spring. Contemplate this myth in the light of your own life – what things will become renewed in your life at the end of winter?

Summing Up

- The past is over. It has educated and enriched you, but it is no place to live your life now – let it go.

- We only live in the present. We cannot predict the future – make today special.

- Practise the art of mindfulness – even the most mundane tasks will take on a new meaning.

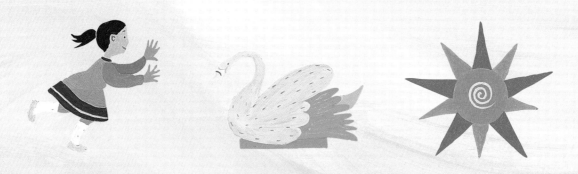

- Let the beauty and wonder of nature soothe your ills and refresh your spirit.

- Live in harmony with the seasons. Allow the energy of spring and the retreat of winter to nourish your soul.

- Gather the harvest of all the good in your life. Give gifts of appreciation to all your friends and loved ones.

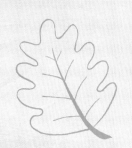
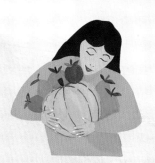
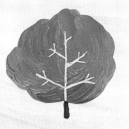

The Eye of the Storm

Even in the fiercest hurricane there is a calm, silent centre –
the eye of the storm. We can take inspiration from this by
learning to appreciate the serenity and tranquillity in the
centre of our being. As our responsibilities, problems and
concerns whirl around us, sometimes threatening to knock
us off balance, we are warmed and comforted by our inner
serenity and profound sense of peace. Through the vehicle
of this inner tranquillity we are able to face our fears with
confidence, nurture our relationships and build strong,
healthy ties with our friends and families, and to face
courageously the difficult times brought about through loss.
What is more, when we send our peace out into the storm,
we can quiet the tempest of others, if only for a moment.

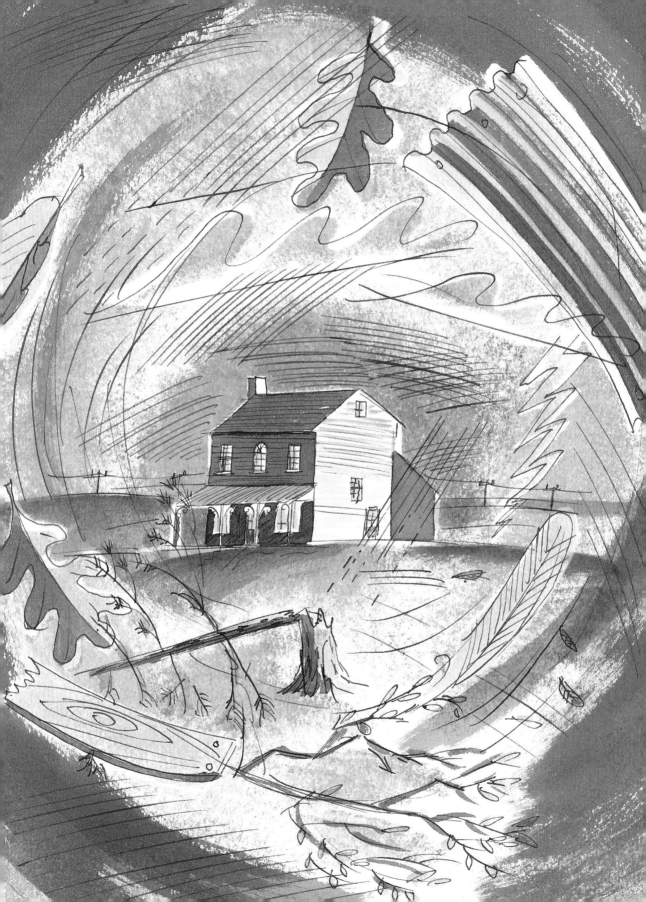

Overcoming Fears

Jawaharlal Nehru, India's first Prime Minister, speculated that "There is perhaps nothing so bad and so dangerous in life as fear." In almost every case of stress, the fear of what may go wrong lies at the heart of the anxiety. If we can successfully combat our fears, relaxation becomes much easier to achieve.

Our fears may be specific, such as a fear of flying or of spiders, or general – an all pervading sense of anxiety that has been present for so long that we can't determine its cause. Whatever the root of our fear, taking steps to control the immediate symptoms permits us to find the clarity and confidence we need to tackle its cause and free ourselves from its world for ever. When the familiar feelings of panic emerge, take steps to calm yourself. Concentrate on your breathing, and try to slow it down. Pay attention as you breathe out, making it as slow and graceful as you can; breathe in one long action. This will give you an immediate sense of peace. Try repeating a phrase, or *mantra*, to yourself, such as the word "strength" or the phrase "I am not afraid, I am at peace." As you do this the mantra's vibrations will penetrate your mind and fill you with feelings of calm.

When we have to face a particular, unknown situation we often feel at our most nervous. For example, we may feel anxious before making a speech in front of a large group of people. But if we can prepare ourselves emotionally, the event will seem less daunting. Begin by taking some slow, deep breaths. Close your eyes, and in your mind, imagine the day of your speech. Look at the crowd waiting expectantly for you to begin. Hear them chatting among themselves. Look at the stage, it seems alarmingly empty and large. You will probably find familiar flutterings rising in your stomach, your heart rate may speed up or your palms become sticky. Notice these feelings, but do not worry

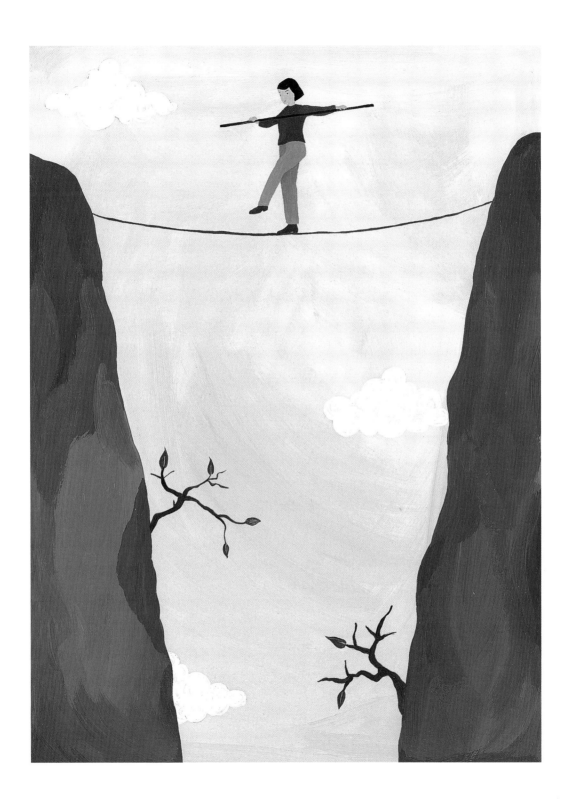

about them. Pretend that you are the type of person for whom fear is unknown. You are completely in control and sure of your success. Picture yourself dressed smartly and perfectly prepared to give a scintillating speech. You stride out onto the stage, and such is your presence that the audience hum instantly quietens. As you talk they hang on every word. Gaze toward them as if they were supportive friends, rather than critical strangers. As you finish you are greeted with loud, enthusiastic applause. If you repeat this scene in your mind several times in the run-up to the real occasion, on the day the all-pervading sense of fear will be gone.

When our fears are less specific, we can deal only with the symptoms. In a cool dark room, relax and close your eyes. Take a few deep breaths, and, as you do so, imagine calming deep blue air filling your lungs and permeating your body. Each time you breathe in, more blue air enters your lungs and as it does so, you feel more and more relaxed. After a few minutes, begin a visualization. You are in a large field. In front of you is an enormous hot air balloon. It is tethered to the ground with strong ropes. Attached to the balloon is a large straw basket. You walk up to it, and in the basket you place all your nervous emotions – the fluttering feeling in your stomach, the shakiness of your hands and the dryness in your mouth. Keep filling the basket until all your symptoms have disappeared and the basket is full. Move around the balloon and untie each rope. The balloon begins to rise and you watch it as it travels far away, until it is only a small dot in the sky. All your nervousness has gone with it. Take a few more deep breaths as you look at the clear blue sky – fear and negativity have disappeared into the far beyond. As you breathe in and out, pure, crisp white air fills your lungs, replacing all your fears with confidence.

Take to the Skies

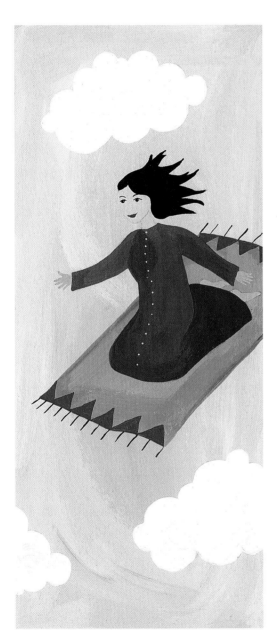

Air travel is said to be 25 times safer than car travel, but fear of flying (aerophobia) is one of the most commonly held fears of all. Can you identify what you are afraid of? Does it stem from a real experience, or from your imagination? What is your worst fear – the risk of engine trouble or pilot error? Is take-off, landing or turbulence more disturbing than other times in the flight?

We can read about flying and its safety statistics and enroll on a fear of flying course, but in many cases, if we can identify the trigger (is it the moment you make the booking? at check-in? as you wait in your seat for take-off?), we can pre-empt our habitual reactions to flying and prepare ourselves to take off in confidence.

Visualize the moment that your fear begins to build. Recall it in as much detail as possible. If it is the moment you check in, watch yourself approach the desk. What does the attendant behind the desk look like? What questions are you asked? As you feel your anxiety rise, imagine breathing it out and replacing it with an in-breath of calm. Repeat the visualization regularly in the days before you fly and try to transform your habitually fearful reaction into a calm one.

Making Peace with Our Emotions

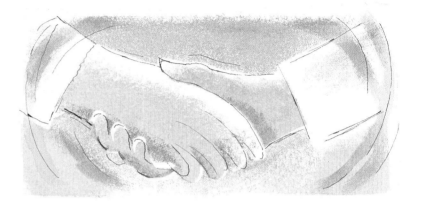

Strong feelings can be all-consuming. At least once in our lives we are gripped by fear, swept away by love, or consumed by sadness. When we are not aware of their strength, our emotions have the power to make us forget our inner peace and pull us into the thick of the storm. Cultivating our awareness of the power that lies in every emotion, allows us to experience, say, the joys and sadnesses of life without being governed by them – while they whirl around in the cyclone, we can remain dispassionate and calm in the centre.

Some emotions, particularly negative ones such as anger or jealousy, can be hard to control – we need to expel them. The next time you feel, say, anger or envy building up you might try writing a letter to an imaginary friend – or even to yourself. Explain all the negative emotions that you feel – be as frank as you can. Then read over what you have written, take a deep breath, tear up the letter and throw it away. Now write yourself another letter highlighting all the wonderful things in your life – the love of a partner, the beauty of your children, the fulfilment in your work and the support of your friends. Read over this letter too, but don't tear it up. Put it in a safe drawer – and refer to it whenever you feel destructive emotions welling up.

Dousing the Flames

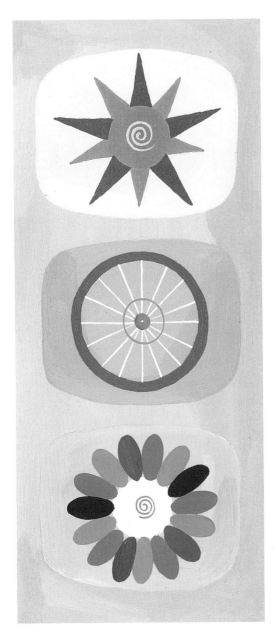

Think about how refreshing it feels to wake in the middle of the night and hear gentle raindrops pattering against the window. After a dry spell the rain seems to cleanse our spirits and calm our busy minds. We can draw upon this natural, healing power of water in times of emotional turmoil.

Perhaps the most commonly used metaphor for the emotions is fire – for example, we talk of the flames of passion, burning desire and the raging fire of anger. A good way to douse the flames of emotion is simply to take a few moments to be alone. Close your eyes and think about how you feel. Visualize your emotions using the metaphor of fire. Your anger may be a scorching inferno; your grief a circle of flames around you; your emotional pain some smouldering coals in the grate. Take some deep breaths and imagine a shower of soothing fresh rain gently washing your body and spirit. As it rains the fires go out – steam rises and then disappears for ever, taking with it your self-consuming emotions. You are released from the power of your emotions and can deal with the causes of your deep feelings more rationally and calmly.

Harmonious Union

Find a watchword

Disagreements occur in the most loving of partnerships. During an argument, we sometimes say things we regret, or let loose a number of frustrations that have nothing to do with the issue at hand. To avoid this it may be helpful to devise a watchword with your partner. Saying a word such as "stop", "calm", or "love" during an argument can be a prompt to stop rowing for long enough to let heated emotions settle. During a relaxing time with your partner, decide what your watchword will be. How will you react to it during an argument? For example, you could stop arguing, hold hands and spend a silent minute looking into each other's eyes. Once the time is up, you can continue your discussion more calmly.

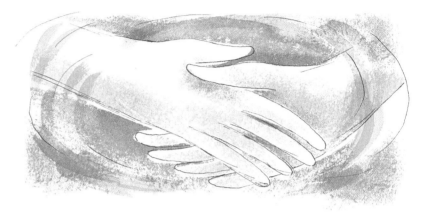

Love may make us feel on top of the world, but it can also make us feel anxious and vulnerable. For most of us, a relationship with a life-partner is the most rewarding and fulfilling relationship of all. However, even the most successful of these unions experience periods of difficulty, throwing up some of the most complex and agonizing emotions in life. At their best relationships provide us with happiness, support, security and fulfilment.

Although this is certainly not true for all cases, many common relationship problems, such as over-sensitivity, jealousy or fear of rejection, stem from one or other partner's lack of self-esteem. In order to get the very best out of our relationships, through both good times and bad, we need to be at ease with who we are, and to believe that we are worthy of our partner's love. Try the following visualization to build your belief in the importance that you have in your partner's life. Lie down in a dark, quiet room. Close your eyes and breathe deeply, let all your tension float away with each out-breath. Imagine that in the centre of your chest is a beautiful pink rosebud. Think about how much love you have for your partner and the love he or she, in turn, extends toward you. Imagine that the inner light of your own love is the source of energy for the rose. Visualize your love enveloping the flower. As it does so, each petal unfurls. The open rose sends out a beautiful scent and a rosy, pink glow. Just as you have given love through your own inner light, the rose sends its own loving light back to you.

The time we spend alone with our partner is precious. Making the most of it in terms of both physical and emotional communication is paramount for a stress-free relationship. Taking a bath together is a wonderful way of soothing tense muscles and promoting a deep sense of intimacy. Prepare the room by lighting candles and playing soft, relaxing music. Run a warm bath and add scented essential oils, such as rose oil, which opens the heart and emotions; sandalwood, which relaxes the body and stimulates desire; and ylang-ylang or jasmine, both of which are aphrodisiacs. As you both relax in the bath, talk about happy memories, future plans and your love for each other. Avoid discussing topics such as problem children or any other frustrations. You are secure in each other's presence as, together, your stresses melt away.

Although a moment of relaxation is not the time to discuss worries, it is important to share the bad as well as the good times in a partnership. If we make it a habit to discuss our needs and problems with each other, our relationship becomes more open, honest and fulfilling. Set aside an appropriate time for discussion, for example early evening, and talk in a neutral place, such as a dining room or kitchen, but not the bedroom. Don't discuss problems when you are feeling tired or stressed, and avoid using a room where you usually relax. During your conversation, try to keep to the topic in hand, rather than diverting attention toward other issues. Be honest but stop to consider your partner's emotions as well as your own as you state your case. It may be frightening to expose strong or negative feelings to a partner, but as you work through your problems together, your bond is reaffirmed. Emotional honesty is essential in maintaining a successful relationship. Once you have reached a conclusion, clear the air both literally and figuratively. Reaffirm your love for your partner, and open the windows in the room to let clean, fresh air blow the tension away.

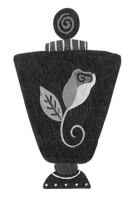

Between the Generations

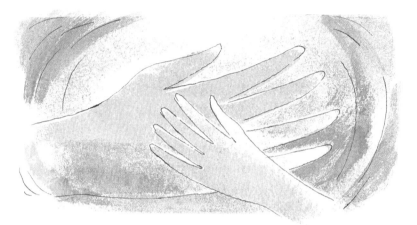

The home we make for our families, as much as it is a place of security and comfort, is a place of learning and creativity – where children learn about morality, sociability, interaction, relationships and most importantly themselves. With all that creative energy being channelled into forming individuality, is it any wonder that family conflicts occur?

The relationships we have with our children when they are small are the most formative of their lives. Try to make sure that you do things as a family at least once a day – perhaps your special time is when you and your partner read a bedtime story with your child. Togetherness helps children to feel secure in the strength of the family bond.

Perhaps some of the most difficult times for a family are teenage years. There are no hard-and-fast rules to apply when our children begin their transformation into adults. As a guide be firm but fair – one set of rules goes for all, including parents. In hard times take support from other parents – almost all teenagers are difficult in some way.

Once we have made it through the emotional turbulence of puberty in the family, we can all emerge stronger and more deeply bonded than ever before. Savour every moment with your children – before you know it they may have children of their own.

A Child's Wisdom

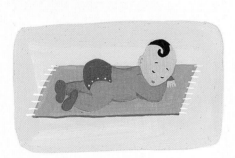

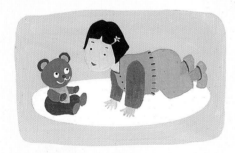

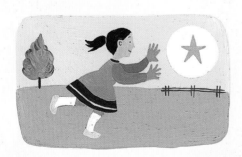

As adults, we learn through habit or example to reject much of the direct, uncompromising view of the world we had as children. Instead of experiencing challenges with wonder and curiosity, we tend to shy away, afraid of the chaos they may cause or perhaps even the financial expense.

But, by experiencing the world with a child's wisdom, with trust, curiosity and energy, we can lose some of the cynicism that adulthood will have taught us. Allow yourself to trust your partner and loved ones unconditionally. This will encourage joy, openness and honesty between you – an enriching and rewarding aim.

For a child the world is filled with wonder. Try exploring a new part of town, or allow an entirely new subject to fill you with passion. Practise finding magic in everyday things. Think, when you break open an egg for your breakfast, now you are the first person ever to see inside!

The energy and vitality of children can be exhausting for a parent. But try adopting such an enthusiasm for life for yourself. As you throw yourself into activities and work, you will find that you achieve more, and find it easier to relax and sleep when you are done.

Extended Circles

Good relations

We often take the support of our family and friends for granted, particularly during times of stress. Taking the time to say thank you to family members and friends for their support, openly displaying our affection toward them, and giving them presents are all ways of expressing appreciation and reinvigorating and reaffirming our relationships. Set aside half an hour each week to consider the benefits you have received from your family or your friends over the course of the last week. Picture each person in your mind, try to quantify how they have helped you, even if you haven't seen or spoken to them. What might they have taught you in the past that you called upon during recent times? Mentally thank them for their support. If you can, make an effort to thank them personally, too.

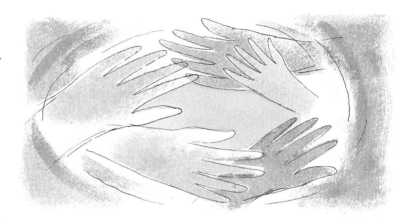

Since the beginning of time, we have relied upon our families for protection, emotional warmth and companionship. Under the safe canopy of the family unit, we learn communication skills, sociability, honesty, sharing, assertion and countless other life-tools. In short, our families give us the social training we need so that we can function in the community later on, as adults.

The bonds of the immediate family are to be cherished and nurtured. Try to spend days together as often as you can, delighting in an activity you all enjoy. It could be a sport, such as horse-riding or swimming, or a sightseeing trip or simply a picnic in a local park. Enjoying leisure time together creates wonderful shared memories – ones that provide an indelible link between all of you and encourage positive interaction beyond the confines of your family home.

Although we may spend the majority of our time with our immediate relations, many of us also have grandparents, uncles, aunts, cousins and so on. Some family members may live far away, some of whom we may never have met. Even so, we are joined to them by a common bond. During a relaxation time, close your eyes and imagine the love that connects all your family members together as an unbreakable white strand of light. It is a bond of love that will provide support and comfort for every family member throughout his or her life. See the strand of light forming a web, like a safety net, as it extends to the members of your household, to your parents and siblings, and on to more distant family members. You may find your family's imaginary web of love stretches to far-flung places extending over thousands of miles. Draw strength from the fact that, wherever you are and whatever happens to you, your family network will reach out to protect you.

Of course, for many of us, particularly in the West, our friends supply the immediate network of support in our day-to-day lives. Most of us find that developing a friendship out of an acquaintance is a gradual process. Just like romantic relationships, an open heart, respect for others and generosity with our time will bring friends into our lives. Spend some time meditating on the value of your friends. What emotional gifts did they bring to you when you first met them? It may have been friendly companionship on the first day of school, or they may have been a fellow enthusiast for a new sport. How have your friends changed your life? How have you changed your friends' lives? What have you discovered together?

We can never have too many friends. By extending the hand of friendship, we can always discover new sources of love, affection, happiness and companionship – all of which help us to weather the most fierce of emotional storms. The thoughts we send out to people and the actions we take toward them often have a profound effect on how others deal with us. Practise sending out messages of goodness to all the people around you – from the stranger next to you on the train to work, to a new mother at your child's kindergarten. Don't forget those for whom you don't care initially, such as the angry driver who honks at you in a traffic jam or the surly shop assistant. A smile or a kind word can diffuse a bad atmosphere, and could even be the start of a fulfilling relationship. New friends and acquaintances help you to push out the boundaries of your "comfort zone", and increase your resources of support and happiness.

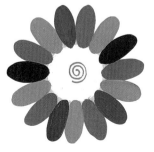

Growing through Loss

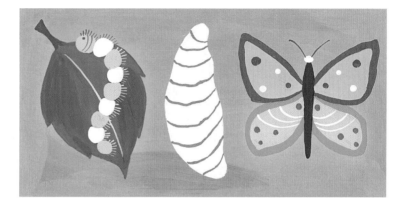

Loss, in its broadest sense, can take many forms: separation, divorce, leaving home or redundancy. However, the most devastating loss that any of us has to cope with is the death of a loved one. Bereavement is a source of profound stress. It can affect all aspects of our lives: our appetite may seem to disappear; sleep may become elusive or erratic; concentration may seem impossible; and relaxation or laughter the things furthest from our minds. As a result we may lose a sense of ourselves, feel vulnerable and develop a dread for the future. Grief shakes our ability to cope and increases our susceptibility to illness.

It can be almost impossible to predict how any of us will grieve. But psychologists have identified a typical pattern for our emotions during such a difficult time. First of all we feel shocked and, quite probably, numb (this in itself can add to the distress – we may begin to feel guilty that the emotions we expect seem unforthcoming). Then, usually after a few days or weeks, we move on to feelings of disbelief, denial, helplessness, anger and, finally, acceptance. These stages of mourning cannot be rushed or denied. By living through them we give ourselves time for emotional healing and adjustment.

Perhaps one of the most difficult things to come to terms with at the death of a loved one is how our own emotions – the love we have for that person – go on, and yet the recipient is no longer there to receive them. Many of us struggle with this concept, and try to sever ourselves from our feelings of love. But we may find it easier to keep alive that loving bond. Try visualizing the loving connection that still exists between you and the person you have lost. You may think of it as a rope tying you together with one end disappearing into the distance. If you shake the rope the vibrations of your love ripple along the connection until the rope goes out of sight. Imagine, moments later, a vibration coming back to you. The bond of love and the communication of that love is eternal. There's no need to hurt ourselves by trying to cut ourselves off, because our love is always there.

Many of us who long for a reunion with our loved one find solace in spiritual belief. The notion of an afterlife can be extremely comforting, and we can also seek consolation through prayer or meditation. During such practices, we can visualize the departed in our minds – we can speak to them, tell them of our feelings or just talk about our lives and the most recent events, just as we did when the person was alive. We may even be able to imagine the answers we receive in return. We needn't hold to any particular religious belief to do this – a spiritual conversation can benefit us all.

If you feel that there are things left unsaid between you and your loved one, why not try writing a letter to them, setting the record straight? Express your hurt or feelings of guilt. Tell them how much you love and miss them. Even though many of us might find this exercise distressing, it provides us with a release – by writing down our thoughts, we move them outside our minds where they can be let go, helping us find a small, inner pocket of calm in which to find peace.

After the shock of bereavement has subsided, we can find ways to celebrate the deceased's life – plant a beautiful tree, take a journey of remembrance, or simply light a candle in memory. Even though we will always feel a sense of loss, the wrenching pain of raw grief will fade and we will find calm as we emerge into a new future.

Healing the Self

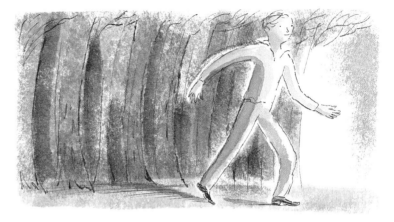

Facing up to ill health – minor or major – is an important part of leading a relaxed lifestyle. If we are worried about illness, we need to tackle our concerns head on. We might decide to take steps to improve our lifestyle and become more aware of our body's needs, perhaps through eating regularly and more healthily, taking regular exercise, resting properly, and so on. We also need to make sure that our minds are healthy – physical and mental health are mutually dependable and your body will give out physical warning signs when our minds are feeling out of sorts. Likewise, we may find that we become temperamental or argumentative, or we may find it hard to concentrate, when our physical self is not working at peak efficiency.

Of course, if we actually feel unwell, we should see a doctor. One of the most extraordinary things about how we treat our bodies is illustrated by comparison with how we treat other vehicles in our lives. If we hear an unusual knocking sound in our car, we take the car straight to the garage to get it checked out. But if our bodies develop an unusual "knocking" (a warning sign), we keep pushing them, until eventually something breaks and we are forced to do something about it. In fact, our bodies deserve at least the same respect as our cars: nothing is more important than our well-being. Statistics show that men in particular tend to ignore the "knocking sounds" of ill-health (such as headaches, unexplained pains, excessive tiredness, loss of appetite, and even pimples). But all of us, when faced with the possibility of illness, find that our fears about the meanings of any warning signs often get the better of us (even if, in our hearts, we suspect that those fears are unfounded). If we do not face up to and review any potential problems, we only make ourselves feel miserable (the possibility of illness weighs heavily in our minds) and as a consequence we become still more susceptible to bad health.

If you have a health concern, seek advice from a professional as soon as you can. Even if your fears turn out to be well-founded, most conditions are more effectively treated if they are detected early. At the very least, talk things through with someone close to you – a friend's advice is no substitute for professional medical advice, but you will have aired your concerns, and given yourself the opportunity to view them objectively through the eyes of another person.

Minor illness, although it may not seem like it, does have its benefits. If we come down with a cold or a migraine, say, our body is telling us to stop and to take a rest. Although it is the body's desperate defence mechanism against stress, illness forces us to take time out. So, when you feel ill, don't go rushing back to work because you think that the office cannot cope without you for another day or so: allow yourself plenty of time to recover. In our frenetic lives, we often ignore the need for convalescence, but, in fact, it is an invaluable opportunity to let our bodies complete the healing process.

Bring the spirit of convalescence into your life – after any illness, or even after a period of great stress, take things easy for a week or two. If you cannot take time off work, at least try not to take on too much responsibility, and spend plenty of time relaxing with your loved ones at home at the weekends and in the evenings. If you can take time off, take a holiday. You owe it to your body to keep it well and listen to what it tells you – it is after all the most precious vehicle you own.

Emotional help

The onset of a serious illness or emotional breakdown is a source of enormous stress. More than ever relaxation is important. It allows us a chance of healing. Our emotions and feelings may be so strong, or even violent, that our friends and family, although loving, are ill-equipped to help us. Support groups or self-help organizations can provide us with unique opportunities to share our worries with others who sympathize, and gain useful advice. A counsellor will help us to see our lives in a new light and understand our confusing emotions more clearly. Without fear of rebuff, we can explore our deepest and most painful feelings. With a counsellor's help, we can reach our own solutions and act on them.

Summing Up

- After a loss, devastating as it may be, look into the fabric of your life, and reassess your aims and ambitions.

- Your family and friends will give you peaceful sanctuary in the midst of chaos.

- Learn from the wisdom of children – look at the bright side of life and truly live in the moment.

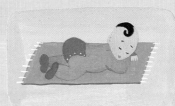
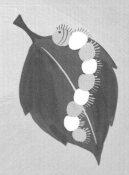

• Trust in the permanence of love, it will nourish and support you for ever – even when loved ones are gone.

• Maintaining your physical health, even during periods of emotional disquiet, keeps you focused. Look after yourself.

• When difficult times arise with a partner, communicate.

 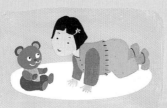 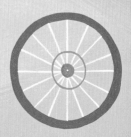

Work Hard, Play Hard

Western society tends to lay great emphasis on competition and success. Consequently, many of us feel under increasing pressure to perform perfectly in all facets of our lives. But none of us is perfect, and although we may wish to do our best at everything, we should try not to burden ourselves with the task of being all things to all people as well as to ourselves. The truth is that nothing lies beyond our grasp, but our hands are too small to hold simultaneously all that we can reach. Keeping work and home separate is paramount for optimum relaxation. Simple rules, such as leaving work at work and family life at home, can be hard to live by — especially in a world of portable computers and mobile telephones. In this chapter we look at ways to make these two important parts of our lives as easy on each other — and on us — as possible.

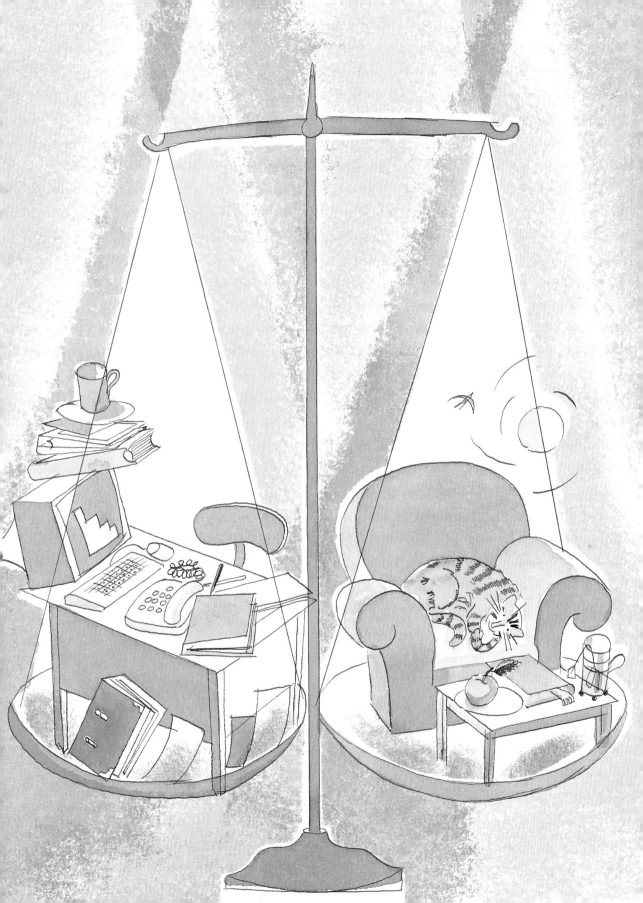

Workplace Worries

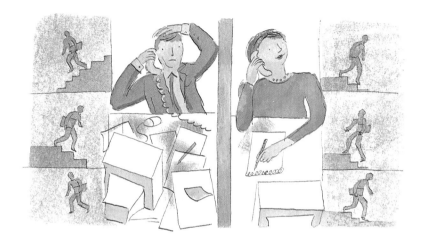

Our jobs can be a source of great satisfaction and self-esteem, giving us a sense of achievement and pride as well as an income. The workplace can be a place of opportunity in which we learn and develop our skills with enthusiasm. On the other hand, for many people work is a primary source of disquiet. Long working hours have meant that finding time to unwind is increasingly rare. Try a little review of your working day now – it will indicate whether or not you are giving too much to your work. How many hours do you work each day? Do you skip meals (probably lunch or breakfast) because you feel that they waste valuable working time? What time do you get home? How long do you spend unwinding before going to bed, and what do you do to unwind?

Most of us are unable to change easily our working environment or the work-ethic of our jobs. The onus, therefore, falls on us to adapt, plan and *make* time where schedules might indicate there is none. Keeping hold of our priorities is an important key to relaxation with regard to work – and we should never place such importance on a work issue that our partner or child takes second place.

Another key is thinking positively about our work. Whatever job we do, it gives us some benefits. Our wages help us maintain a standard of living. Our work colleagues provide us with companionship. Work provides a structure for our lives – if nothing else, making us appreciate the fun we have on vacation! Spend a few moments contemplating the positive aspects of your job. Now consider your worries. Are your deadlines consistently tight? Is your workload too heavy, and your resources too stretched? Does your lack of autonomy make you feel unimportant? Do you frequently disagree with your boss or colleagues? Are you a victim of bullying, racism or sexism? As you list your concerns, think about how you could change each situation. Is there a sympathetic manager you could discuss your issues with? Could you delegate to lessen your load? You may be surprised at what you can achieve to remedy your situation once you have defined the problems.

Giving ourselves a routine to work by helps us to define our achievements, and to leave work behind with satisfaction at the end of each day. Before each working day begins, find a quiet place (even if this turns out to be the restroom!) and make a list of all the things you need to get done. Number your list in order of priority. Try not to fall into the trap of thinking that every single item is as important as the next – force yourself to prioritize. Back at your post, you can begin your day with a clear head, working from the most important item to the least. Although unforeseen problems can crop up on any day and your routine may be interrupted, the list will give you focus. Once you have dealt with the unexpected, you will have something to turn your mind back to – the break in your working rhythm will have been a minor disruption, not a complete disaster for your powers of concentration. If you have not completed all the items at the end of the day, be reasonable about how much extra time you spend at work: the items that were least important today can become the priorities tomorrow. You will undertake them fresh and relaxed, probably completing them more efficiently than you would if you had slaved away late into the evening during time that should be for leisure.

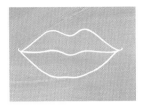

Balancing the books

Our choice of leisure activities can help us to become more productive in our working lives. If we ensure that our leisure and work provide us with true variety in life, we can take another step to beating stress. For example, competitive and goal-driven jobs, such as sales or marketing, can be balanced with an uncompetitive pastime such as yoga, or a creative task such as painting. However, less competitive jobs (but among the most stressful), such as working on a factory production line, may be better contrasted with highly stimulating pastimes, such as learning a foreign language or taking up a competitive or team sport.

Working Together

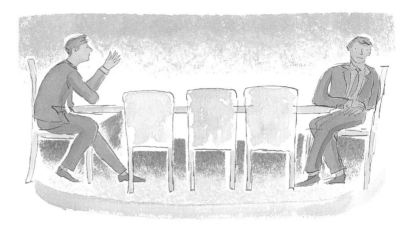

We spend a great deal of time in the company of our workmates. Our relationships with colleagues may be some of the most enduring, satisfying and close encounters in our lives. When we trust our fellow workers, we gain a positive, new dimension to our work. However, inevitably in a place where not all (if any) of our co-workers are of our own choosing, personalities will clash and tensions surface.

No matter what difficulties arise between you and another colleague, at work we have common goals. We all want to succeed, but our success depends equally upon others as it does upon ourselves. If one team member shines, then so does the team; if all team members shine, then the possibilities for success soar. Learn to be assertive (see opposite) but not aggressive in making your point heard; learn to listen and respond rather than to react. Extend the hand of friendship when things don't go your way as well as when they do and try not to make rash judgments about people. Take a difficult colleague aside to discuss a possible solution to any problems. And remember that the more positive energy you send out, the more positive energy you will get back.

Making Yourself Heard

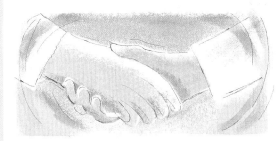

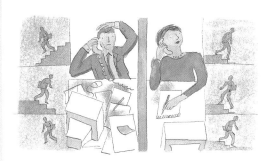

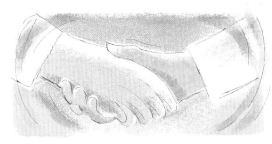

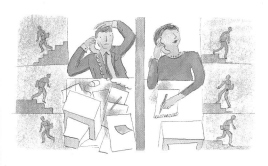

To work best with our colleagues we need to communicate effectively and efficiently with them. By assertively expressing our requirements, and being honest about our strengths and limitations, we will undoubtedly reduce our stress at work. The following technique is one which can be used to make sure that our voice is heard in any situation, even those outside work.

If you know that you are going to have a difficult conversation or meeting, run over the most important points you want to make the night before. Write them down and read them over several times. Now, imagine that as you make each point, it hits a brick wall and comes bouncing back at you. Take a deep breath and send it back with a calm and consistent movement. Each time the point makes contact with the wall it knocks out a brick until, finally, the wall disappears. During the actual meeting, whatever is thrown at you should not deter you from making yourself heard and gaining answers to your questions. Articulate your thoughts clearly and concisely. Of course, you can compromise, but never forget your promises to yourself – the things that are important to you are just as worthy of respect and response as those that are important to others.

Holding Pressures at Bay

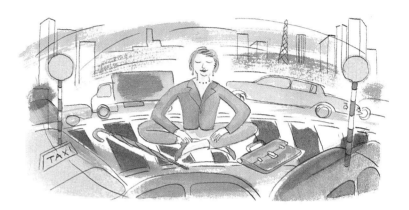

Pressures at work come in a multitude of manifestations, but perhaps the most common problem is a lack of time. We may have to deal with endless meetings, stringent deadlines and a heavy workload every day. Even though we plan our priorities and set ourselves achievable goals, we may still feel that there are not enough hours in the day.

If you feel that you are running out of time at the approach of a deadline, or an urgent problem at home threatens to make you late for an important meeting, first make a conscious effort to calm down. Say "stop" out loud and take a break from your anxiety. Close your eyes and breathe deeply and slowly. Relax your shoulders and notice any symptoms of panic you are feeling. Is your heart beating far too fast? Are your hands shaking or clammy? As you breathe slowly in and out, imagine that time is expanding. If you are focused and calm, time will seem to expand to give you as much as you need to complete your tasks; or as long as you arrive at the meeting calm and collected (ready with a genuine, but confident, apology), those present will think none the less of you. Observe how relaxed your body feels as a result of these realizations – suddenly time no longer seems your enemy.

Exercise 16
Acupressure for Relieving Tension

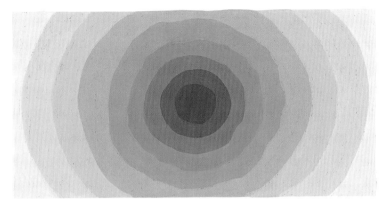

According to Chinese theory, stress is caused when our flow of qi, or life energy (see p.15), is blocked or reduced. The Chinese therapy of acupressure teaches that we can apply pressure to special points on our skin to unblock qi. These subtle techniques can bring instant relief at any time.

• If tension is making you feel nauseous, press your thumb firmly between the two bones on your inner forearm, three fingers' width below the wrist crease. Hold your thumb there for 30–60 seconds and then swap thumbs to press on the other arm.

• A tension headache can be soothed by massaging the web between your thumb and first finger. Use the opposite hand to press as close as possible to the point where the two bones meet. Continue massaging for about a minute and then repeat on the other hand.

• To help relieve anxiety and feelings of panic or extreme pressure, find the spot one finger's width below the crease on the inside of your wrist. Press your thumb on the skin directly in line with your little finger. Hold the pressure for around a minute or until you feel calm.

Learning to Switch Off

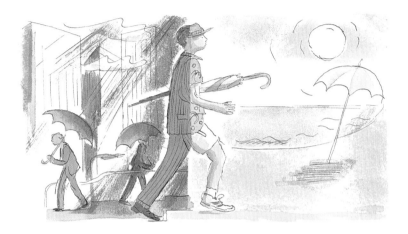

Many of us find it difficult to maintain a healthy balance between our careers and home lives. We may take work home or find it difficult to stop thinking about work-related problems while resting. Inevitably, this has a damaging effect on our personal lives. It is also counterproductive – if the time were spent relaxing instead, we would return to work refreshed, energetic and able to give it our full attention.

Imagine your life is contained within a series of boxes. In one is your work, another contains your leisure, in yet another is your close family and so on. Our lives are so rich that we all have hundreds of boxes, each neatly holding an aspect of our lives. As we finish our work for the day, we can place all our work issues in the relevant container and close the lid until the next day. Similarly, after our children have gone to bed, we can focus our attention on our partner. Separating the different aspects keeps us free to move on unencumbered by other issues. However, if a box overflows and its contents begin to mingle with the contents of other boxes, we soon lose our ability to concentrate fully on anything and we are vulnerable to stress.

To help keep your activities in the proper boxes, find small routines that help you delineate your life. As you prepare for work, imagine you are performing a ceremony, designed to focus your mind on your job. Your early morning relaxation or meditation, putting on your clothes, brushing your hair, eating breakfast and travelling to work make you ready for the start of the working day. By the time you arrive at your workplace, you are fully focused on the day's tasks.

At the end of a working day, think about your achievements. However small they seem, they provide us with a sense of fulfilment – of having finished. Then, tidy your desk or work space, so it is uncluttered when your return. Psychologically, this will help you to feel that the day is done. If you work from home, make sure that at a certain time you clear away your working area and, if possible, shut the door to the room. Don't go back in there until the morning.

Many of us face stressful journeys home from work. We may have to endure overcrowded and unreliable public transport or the frustration of being stuck in traffic jams. But even this time can be used for relaxation. On a bus or train, read a good book or the newspaper (avoiding any article that may relate to your job – save those for the morning). Play some soothing music in the car, or ask your children to make you a special coming-home cassette (they might choose the songs to go onto it, sing on it themselves, or mix music with messages for you). Try a visualization. Imagine that you are in a small sailing boat, moored to a jetty. The sun is shining and you can't wait to leave and travel toward your family and friends. However, the boat is weighed down with many bulky, heavy packages, which represent your workday worries. You can't untie the boat because the rope is straining against the weight. One by one, you heave the packages onto the shore, stacking them up ready to be dealt with the next day. As you do so the boat becomes lighter, and you can easily untie the rope. Leaving your worries behind, you sail off toward home through a beautiful, calm sea.

The inner smile

A Chinese technique called the "inner smile" is a quick way to switch off. At the end of the working day, sit comfortably with your back straight and your arms relaxed at your sides. Think about something that amuses you. Allow yourself to smile – internally if you prefer. Let the smile shine all over your face and glisten in your eyes. Then imagine that it travels inward to spread through your body. As your smile radiates within and without, notice the feeling of relaxation and calm that it generates. Now all is well with your inner self, you can return home and enjoy the rest of the day to the full.

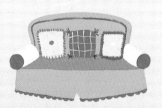

Relaxing at Home

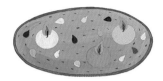

Just as animals retreat to places of warmth and security during illness or when raising a family, so we need a home as a stable base for our lives. Our home is more than just a shelter – it is our sanctuary from the world. Here, we can be truly ourselves: we can relax, plan, express ourselves openly and shake off our cares.

In most houses or flats, each room has a designated purpose – the kitchen is where we cook, the living room where we relax, the bedroom where we sleep, and so on. However, often we merge the functions – perhaps we don't have a dining room so we eat in the lounge, or we don't have a study so we work in the bedroom. Just as we compartmentalize our lives in order to relax, we should clearly define the functions of each room in our homes so that, even if we don't have "enough" rooms, space is designated to certain tasks or functions. This enables us to order our lives without the conflicting energies of different kinds of purpose causing us disquiet. If you need some space to work in, but do not have a study, choose part of the house which is dedicated to activity anyway, perhaps the kitchen if there is space for a table or a clear work surface. Although it is not ideal, you could section off a corner of the living room or dining room for work. Try not to use your bedroom as a study – some sleep experts believe that it can disrupt our rest. If you have guests staying over, but do not have a spare room in which they can sleep, screen off part of the living room before they arrive. It is important for guests to feel that they have their own space. This will also separate the sleeping space from the space dedicated to communication, so that when your guests go to bed the room will not be buzzing with talkative energy. Even better, try to move the evening's entertainment to another place (say, the dining room or garden) to keep the living room tranquil for your guests' sleep.

Positive Energy in the Home

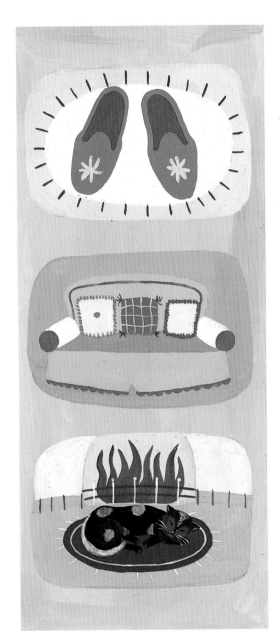

We have all entered a house and felt inexplicably ill-at-ease, and we have all been in homes that instantly feel warm and welcoming. Everyone's home contains energy from its past and present inhabitants.

Laughter, happiness, relaxation and love in a home will imbue it with plenty of positive vibrations – your home will feel joyous to return to and comforting and peaceful when you are there. However, if your home seems unwelcoming, or you find yourself overcome with fatigue, depression or you are prone to illness when there, clearing your space of negative vibrations and filling it with positive energy will help you to relax and turn your home into a haven of peace.

Give the entire house a spring clean: clear out dust and cobwebs from far flung corners – such as the attic, cellar or garage – as well as visible surfaces. Repaint in colours that inspire you. Fill the house with music you enjoy. Open windows to cleanse the air and fill the home with freshness.

When you move into a new home, clear the old vibrations in preparation for your time there by throwing a housewarming party. This is an old, but effective, tradition of welcoming in new people and making peace with the existing energy.

Once your home is as ordered as possible, walk around the rooms. Stand as near to the centre of each room as furniture allows and close your eyes. Does the atmosphere feel warm or cold? In your mind's eye what colour most suits the room? Where does the sunlight fall during the day and which are the darkest corners? What could you do to make the room feel warmer or calmer? Try to analyze each room in turn and then, over time, set about turning each into a place that (through colour, ornaments or mementos, and furniture) wholly reflects its major purpose. For example, if you were to use colour appropriately, you might paint the living room a relaxing green (this colour reflects nature, so it introduces a sense of harmony and balance in a room). The bedroom might suit a light shade of blue. Far from being a cold colour, pale blue is clean, fresh and calming. The dining room might suit red, which is warm, inviting and sociable. A hallway might suit a vibrant yellow – bestowing vitality and sunny warmth on all those who enter.

Don't be afraid to experiment with colour, and if you feel uncomfortable painting a dark, dimly lit room anything but white, choose cushions of a colour that suits the room, or buy fresh flowers in that colour to place there. Before redecorating, consider the changing light in the room – dimming sunlight and artificial light subtly alter the shades of colours. Buy experimental pots of paint (test pots are available at all good hardware stores) and see what the colour looks like in a dark corner or on a well-lit wall. If a darker shade works better in the sun-exposed areas of a room, think about how you can change the artificial lighting with lamps or candles to brighten naturally darker areas of the room. Add personal touches to family rooms and bedrooms – pictures of happy times together and memorabilia from a vacation keep in mind happy times and create a positive, loving atmosphere.

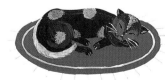

Feng Shui – the Art of Space

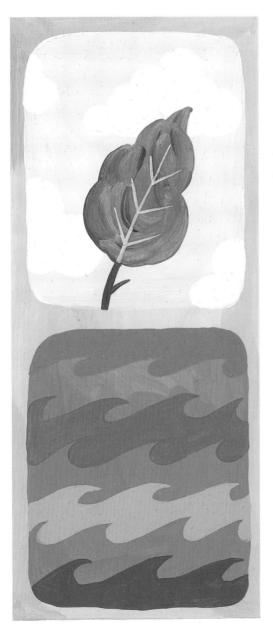

Feng Shui (literally meaning "Wind and Water") is the ancient Chinese art of arranging our living spaces in the most auspicious way and in harmony with the flow of universal energy, qi (see p.15). Originally, the technique was used primarily to discover a prime burial site where the dead might prosper in the next world. Nowadays, however, people in both the East and West use Feng Shui to harmonize their homes.

According to the principles of Feng Shui, clutter impedes the flow of qi: furniture should be well spaced and surfaces clear. Qi is aggravated by sharp pointed objects – spiky plants and angular furniture are not favoured by Feng Shui practitioners. Rounded objects allow qi to flow easily around a room, giving the inhabitants luck, good humour and health.

By stimulating or calming the qi in one area of our home, we can make changes to the part of our lives this room is said to represent. If you wish for a new relationship, for example, light a pair of candles in the southwest corner of the most-frequented room, such as the living room or kitchen. If you feel insecure, you can "ground" yourself by placing a heavy ornament in the most southerly point of the same room.

Vacation Strategies

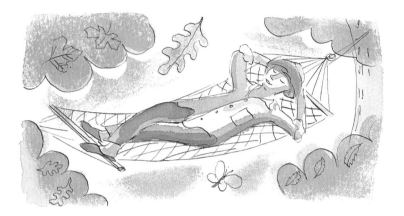

We all know the value of vacations for relaxation. Idyllic thoughts of idling on the beach, exhilarating ski trips or seeing stunning mountain scenery can help to get us through the most difficult and stressful of days, lifting us away from mundane concerns.

Vacations give us the opportunity to rest and replenish our spirit. However, unless we prepare ourselves for a vacation, it can easily become an additional source of stress. This is especially true if we plan to travel or visit somewhere new: the abrupt change in lifestyle may make us feel disoriented, and if we have been under stress, we may even fall ill. For a few days running up to a vacation, try to include more relaxation and meditation into your life. Slow down the pace of what you do each day, so that you can adjust yourself practically, mentally and physically for your forthcoming break. Once you are away, you will be able to abandon all your timetables and routines without a second thought. Although it may be fun to try new activities – learning to dive or ski, or visiting historic monuments – our primary aim should be to relax. However, relaxation manifests itself differently for each of us, so cast off all rules once you are away – do exactly as you please!

Planning a Stress-free Vacation

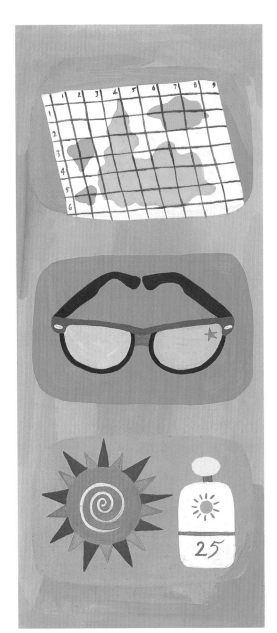

Preparing for a vacation, both practically and mentally, will minimize its potential stress.

Take care of practicalities first. If you are venturing overseas, make sure your passport is valid and you have any relevant visas and had inoculations. Pack plenty of medications, not only prescription ones if you need them, but painkillers, indigestion tablets and insect repellent. Find out as much as you can about your destination before you go and make a note of any activities you want to try or places of interest you wish to visit.

If possible give yourself an extra day to relax before you leave on vacation. If you are used to a pressured lifestyle, you may find it hard to leave the stress behind. Use your extra time to close the door mentally on your problems, so that you begin your vacation with a free heart and tranquil spirit.

As far as possible choose a destination that is as conducive to relaxation as possible. City workers may prefer a break on the coast or in the countryside rather than an urban vacation – even if it is to somewhere as exhilarating as New York or as beautiful as Paris; and an activity vacation such as skiing or hiking may not suit us if we are in need of a rest or if we are generally unfit.

Summing Up

- Give a hundred per cent to your work when you are there, and then forget all about it when you leave.

- Communicate openly with colleagues, so that problems can be dealt with quickly, easily and harmoniously.

- Respect your time and your right to do the best for yourself and your family.

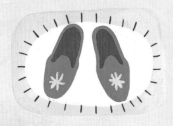 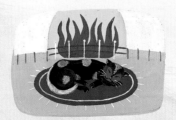 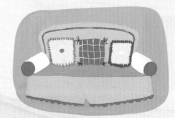

• Plan your vacations. Then, once you are there, take a total break — leave all the worries of home and work behind.

• Try to pursue interests that are different from your job and find balance between work and play.

• Energize your home. Paint it colours that suit you and keep it free from clutter.

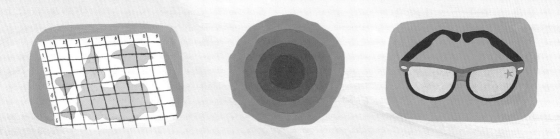

Useful Addresses

US
American Aromatherapy
Association
PO Box 3679
South Pasadena
California 91031

American Holistic Medical
Association
6728 Old Maclain Village
Drive
Maclain
Virginia 22101

American Psychological
Association
750 First Street NE
Washington DC 20002

National Association of
Holistic Aromatherapy
PO Box 76221
Boulder
Colorado

Sivananda Yoga Vendanta
Centre
243 West 24th Street
New York 10011

Stress Education Center
John Mason PhD
315 East Cotati Avenue,
Suite G
Cotati
California 74931

Yoga Research and
Education
PO Box 1386
Lower Lake
California 95457

UK
Clare Maxwell-Hudson
PO Box 457
London NW2 4BR
(for information on
massage courses)

Eastern Clinic
1079 Garratt Lane
Tooting Broadway
London SW17 0LN

The Institute of Optimum
Nutrition
Blades Court
Deodar Road
London SW15 2NU

National Institute of
Medical Herbalists
56 Longbrooke Street
Exeter EX4 6AH

Relaxation for Living
29 Burwood Park Road
Walton on Thames
Surrey KT12 5LH

Yoga for Health Foundation
Ickwell Bury
Biggleswade
Bedfordshire
SG18 9EF

Australia
Biofeedback Meditation
Relaxation Centre
165 Adderton Road
Carlingford
New South Wales 2118

BKS Iyengar Association of
Australia (Yoga)
1 Rickman Avenue
Mosman
New South Wales 2088

Brahma Kumaris Raja Yoga
Meditation Centres of
Australia
Unit 1/307 Glebe Point
Road
Glebe
Sydney 2037

International Federation of
Aromatherapists
1st Floor
390 Burwood Road
Hawthorn
Victoria 3122

International Yoga
Teachers' Association
c/o 14–15 Huddart Avenue
Normanhurst
New South Wales 2076

Maharishi Ayurveda Health
Centres
PO Box 81
Bundoora
Victoria 3083

National Herbalist
Association of Australia
Suite 305, BST House
3 Small Street
Broadway
New South Wales 2007

Canada
Canadian Natural Health
Association
439 Wellington Street
Toronto
Ontario M5V 2H7

Institute of Dynamic
Aromatherapy
Jade Shutes
1983 West 57th Avenue
Vancouver
British Columbia V6P 1T9

L'Institut International du
Stress
659 Hilton Street
Montreal
Quebec H2X 1W6

National Institute of
Nutrition
Suite 302
265 Carling Avenue
Ottawa
Ontario K1S 2E1

Sivananda Yoga Vedanta
Centre
5178 St Lawrene Boulevard
Montreal
Quebec H2T 1R8

Index

Further Reading

ALTERNATIVE MEDICINE

Hill, Clare *The Ancient and Healing Art of Aromatherapy*, Hamlyn (London)

Lawless, Julia *The Illustrated Encyclopedia of Essential Oils*, Element (Rockport, Massachussetts and Dorset, England)

Maxwell–Hudson, Clare *The Complete Book of Massage*, Dorling Kindersley (London and New York)

Tobias, Maxine and John Patrick Sullivan *The Complete Stretching Book*, Dorling Kindersley (London and New York)

EASTERN HEALING

Lam Kam Chuen *Master the Way of Energy*, Fireside (New York)

MacRitchie, James *Chi Kung, Cultivating Personal Energy*, Health Essentials, Element Books (Rockport, Massachussetts and Dorset, England)

Mitchell, Emma *Your Body's Energy*, Macmillan (New York) and Mitchell Beazley (London)

Young, Jacqueline *Acupressure for Health*, Thorsons (London)

MEDITATION

Carrington, Patricia, Ph.D. *The Book of Meditation*, Element Books (Rockport, Massachussetts and Dorset, England)

Fontana, David *The Elements of Meditation*, Element Books (Rockport, Massachussetts and Dorset, England)

Fontana, David *Learn to Meditate*, Chronicle Books (San Francisco) and Duncan Baird Publishers (London)

Shapiro, Eddie and Debbie *Meditation for Inner Peace*, Piatkus (London)

Smith, Erica and Nicholas Wilks *Meditation, a Practical Introduction to the Techniques, the Traditions and the Benefits*, Trafalgar Square (Vermont, Canada)

Walters, J. Donald *Meditation for Starters*, Chrystal Clarity Publishers (Nevada City, California)

RELAXATION

Benson, Herbert *The Relaxation Response*, Avon Books (New York)

George, Mike *Learn to Relax*, Chronicle Books (San Francisco) and Duncan Baird Publishers (London)

Hewitt, James *Teach Yourself Relxation*, Hodder and Stoughton (London)

SELF-CONFIDENCE
Henderson, Julie *The Lover Within*, Station Hill Press (New York)

SLEEP AND DREAMS
ABC of Sleep Disorders, edited by Colin M. Shapiro, Login Brothers Book Company (Chicago)

Fontana, David *The Secret Language of Dreams*, Chronicle Books (San Francisco) and Pavillion Books (London)

Heyneman, Nicholas E., Ph.D. *DreamScape*, Fireside (New York)

Idzikowksi, Chris *The Insomnia Kit*, Eddison Sadd (New York and London)

Hunt, Harry T. *The Multiplicity of Dreams*, Yale University Press (New Haven)

Nicoll, Maurice *Dream Psychology*, Samuel Weiser Inc. (York Beach)

OVERCOMING STRESS
Battison, Toni *Beating Stress*, Macmillan (New York)

Madders, Jane *The Stress and Relaxation Handbook*, Trafalgar Square (Vermont)

Watts, Murray and Professor Gary L. Cooper *Relax: Dealing with Stress*, BBC Books (London)

Wildwood, Chrissie *The Complete Guide to Reducing Stress*, Piatkus (London)

Wilson, Paul *Instant Calm*, Penguin Books (New York and London)

YOGA
Sivananda Yoga Centre *Yoga Mind and Body*, Dorling Kinderlsey (New York and London)

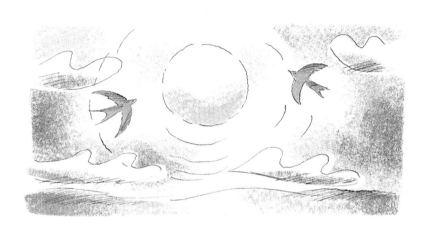